Dear Reader:

In recent years, significant advances in hearing aid technology have dramatically improved the quality of lives for hundreds of thousands of hard of hearing people. Nonetheless, despite the multitude of advanced technological advances and astounding innovation within today's hearing aids, the most important component within the "hearing aid process" is people.

At Oticon our mission is clear. *We strive to help people with hearing loss live the life they want with the hearing they have.* All across our 100+ year history we've sought and received extraordinary input from highly trained researchers, engineers, audiologists, design specialists, psychoacousticians, psychologists, educators, physicians and other professionals.

Perhaps most importantly, we've sought input from the people using our products. These include patients, moms, dads and families—to create the most useful and desirable hearing products possible. Oticon's slogan is "People First" and we take that very seriously to guide us as we create products people want, need and will benefit from.

With similar passion, we're honored to make this abridgement available to you. *The Consumer Handbook on Hearing Loss & Hearing Aids: A Bridge to Healing* (Third Edition) is an easy-to-read, people-based approach to the issues associated with better hearing, hearing loss, hearing aids and assistive technologies. This book isn't about ears or advanced hearing aid technology. It's about people. It's about understanding personal motivations and needs, and it's about listening and learning.

I wish you the very best on your journey to live life maximally with the hearing you have. I believe this book offers common sense and real-world insight into many important issues impacting your journey. As you and your family listen and learn about hearing and hearing loss, I'm confident you'll refer back to this book time and time again as one important bridge to healing.

Sincerely yours,

Peer Lauritsen, President
Oticon Inc.
www.oticonusa.com

Cover concept and development by William Greaves
Concept West, Cave Creek, Arizona

Abridged from
ISBN: 978-0-9661826-9-9

Auricle Ink Publishers
P. O. Box 20607, Sedona AZ 86341
(928) 284-0860
www.hearingproblems.com

Abridged from
The Consumer Handbook on Hearing Loss and Hearing Aids

A Bridge to Healing

REVISED
Third Edition

Richard E. Carmen, Au.D., Editor

Auricle Ink Publishers
Sedona

TABLE OF CONTENTS

CHAPTER ONE
The Emotions of Losing Hearing and a Bridge To Healing

Richard E. Carmen, Au.D.

Dr. Carmen received his Doctor of Audiology Degree from the Arizona School of Health Sciences, a division of the Kirksville College of Osteopathic Medicine. His professional interests have encompassed human studies research, clinical practice and hearing aid dispensing. He has authored or co-authored more than 50 papers, many peer-reviewed, several books and a couple chapters. In addition to writing extensively in the field as a regular contributor to various professional journals and publications, his interest in patient education and consumer awareness has led to a number of articles in such recognized periodicals as *The Saturday Evening Post, Ladies' Home Journal and Self Magazine*. Among many hearing industry board positions over his career, Dr. Carmen remains as one of the technical advisors to The Better Hearing Institute.

Much has changed in hearing aid technology since the second edition of this book (in 2004). Hearing aids have become less obtrusive and they offer superior performance than even a few years ago. With the advent of telecommunication devices such as Bluetooth cell phone receivers, wearing anything in the ear these days is at best passé, and maybe even fashionable. For some, I've noticed that it even seems to be a statement of moving with social change as people talk into thin air presumably using their Bluetooth devices. And yet, if you're like me, sometimes there's that one moment you have to look twice to confirm that you're not observing a schizophrenic on the street simply talking to himself. Then you find yourself saying, "Oh yeah! Oh yeah, he's fine."

What we're seeing here is a sweeping shift in acceptance of "things" worn in or about our ears. You really can no longer tell the difference between telecommunication devices and some state-of-the-art ear-level hearing aids. Some hearing aids are so elegantly designed that they no longer even look like hearing aids, perhaps more closely resembling a piece of jewelry. The results have been profound social change, a shift in thinking by both wearers and observers whereby the stigma of wearing these devices that don't look like hearing aids is essentially gone. At the time of writing of the first and second editions of this book, such a thing was only imagined! While we have virtually transformed social change in less than five years through design, this is not to say all is well on the frontier.

The initial reaction to learning you have hearing loss and must wear hearing aids can still hit you like a brick. (See Appendix I for clarification of degree and types of hearing loss.) By the time a practitioner determines you have hearing loss, you've already been living with it most likely for years, so you're just getting confirmation of what you've already suspected. Even so, for many it's a hard pill to swallow. For some, it rattles them to the core. As Quasimodo, the Hunchback of Notre Dame said in his dying breath as he lay in the arms of the beautiful gypsy girl La Esmeralda, a tear rolling off his cheek, "Why could I not have been made of stone?" His torment reflects that of many of us—the pain of *feeling*.

But feel we must, as this is what characterizes us as human. Emotional experiences may be wonderful, painful, or sometimes perplexing. Yet, more than our physical body, feelings are the substance of our identity. Each of us reacts differently toward the varied experiences of our lives. For centuries, fields of study have been devoted to exploring this fascinating phenomenon, but the search seems to have yielded as much controversy as knowledge. From more than three decades of clinical practice, I've observed some compelling emotions and feelings in my patients. These observations extend into my own family members with loss of hearing, so the feelings we'll be talking about touch home.

I once taught an audiology course in which I had my students wear earplugs for a full day, morning to bedtime. They were asked to log their feelings and emotions and report to the class the following week. We were all overwhelmed by two things: the similarity of their experiences and the depth of their emotions. Students reported they felt inadequate and incompetent. There was also a sense of limitation in areas they'd taken for granted. Simple tasks like using the telephone couldn't be performed without special manipulation, difficulty or strain. Common sounds like ice stirred in a glass, running water or turning a page in a book—sounds that orient us in our environment—were gone.

Driving the car was a new experience. With the absence of wind and traffic sounds, there was a feeling of disorientation. Students quickly realized how important their vision became to compensate for what they could not hear. Yet, such compensation was inadequate. By the end of the day most of the students confessed they were worn out and disturbed by what they had gone through.

"What a horrible experience!" one student remarked.

An apt description I thought.

One student reported she had collapsed into bed crying. Others were unnerved or depressed. Their collective reactions were directly linked to feelings of inadequacy, a deficiency in their daily performance relative to what they expected or how they were accustomed to functioning. Once the earplugs were removed, all ill feelings dissipated. Their sense of normalcy and calm returned. If your significant other has no idea what it feels like to have a hearing loss, this would be an enlightening experience.

While this experiment was useful to normal hearing students, it revealed what you no doubt already know. Hearing is an essential human sense. Its absence would be greatly missed by anyone. As hearing declines, similar to other sensory deficits, we humans have an extraordinary ability to compensate for the loss. Such compensation is a built-in defense mechanism that we give little thought to. It just happens. If you have a heart attack, the body works quickly to establish other pathways and connections. If you lose your sense of smell, your eyes become more probing. When vision diminishes, listening can sharpen. And when hearing declines, you might overcompensate in other ways, also by listening more attentively. Your innate ability to exclude extraneous sounds might kick in. You might cup your hand around your ear. You may find yourself focusing sharply on the speaker, unconsciously observing lip, facial and body movements and gestures. This very natural tendency happens without much conscious awareness. And these things do help you "hear" better. In fact, they work so well that the very act of compensation can fool you into believing that you hear fine. It's for this reason that loss of hearing gives the impression of being so insidious.

"It just kind of crept up on me!" many hard of hearing people confess. Of course it didn't really just creep up.

Something you've probably said many times in your life, and will see repeated, rephrased and reanalyzed in this book is the complaint, "I hear but I don't understand the words clearly!" This is particularly true when trying to communicate in a group, around a few people, or in an environment with background noise such as in a restaurant or automobile. Early on, when you had problems hearing, you may have passed it off as being no more troublesome for you than for anyone else in the same situation. But as issues around poor hearing grew more apparent and the process of communication began breaking down, you must have realized the problem was not going away.

People who develop hearing loss from an explosion, accident, physical trauma or rapidly progressing disease are probably more inclined to deal with it because it is so sudden and unmistakably apparent. But if you're in generally good health and are the type of person who doesn't like to think of yourself as less capable than anyone else, you might have found that you started blaming other people for frequent miscommunication. This is very common. You may think others are not speaking clearly or loudly enough, or they "mumble" their words. It's only when sufficient numbers of people close to you suggest that it's <u>you</u> and not them, that you might have gotten your first inkling of something within your personal communication system has gone awry. Some people never come to this realization and go on believing that others are the source of their communication failure. They continue to blame other people and are discouraged that others appear to enunciate so poorly. Nothing will deteriorate a relationship faster than denial. This is not healthy in any family, and why it's so important to get to the core issues.

Our ego is quite attached to our overall health. Most of us like to think of ourselves as being in shape with a good heart, strong bones, acceptable vision, and good hearing. For some of us, admission of poor hearing is like admitting we've given in to old age. It's like a forced resignation we never invited. The realization of hearing loss places you at a crossroads, offering two quite opposing paths. The first is to admit the hearing loss; the second is to deny it. The former decision (admitting it) allows you to reassess and seek solutions to enhance and maximize your quality of life. The latter decision (denial) negatively impacts every aspect of your life, destroys relationships and decreases your quality of life

To resist the reality of having hearing loss perpetuates miscommunication and the turmoil that goes with it. If we try to ignore loss of hearing, or stop thinking about it, the problem persists. For some people, the crossroads for acknowledging hearing difficulty but doing nothing about it is where they get stuck for years. In fact, the odds are very high that prior to reading this book you've known of your hearing loss for more than five years, during which time frustration, communication problems and hearing difficulties have significantly increased.

Problem-Solving Ground Rules

Before we discuss your feelings about hearing loss, let's first define the terms used and establish the ground rules upon which problems can be solved. "Hearing loss" is the physical condition in your ear. "Hearing difficulties" pertain to specific situations (like trying to hear someone speaking to you). A "hearing problem" is your internalization of the situation, how you process the issues surrounding these situations (like getting upset at your spouse if you miss a word).

These terms are often mistakenly interchanged. If you're in the living room watching television with your family and you realize you're missing too much dialogue, you might ask others in the room if you can turn the volume louder, in which case you think you've solved the hearing difficulty. The reality is your family will object to having the television so loud. This may make you annoyed, or you may feel rejected, angry, resentful, annoyed or other ill feelings—a sure sign of a hearing problem. You're internalizing feelings about a hearing difficulty. As stated earlier, the first step in solving difficulties about your experience is to first acknowledge the challenge, then recognize how you feel about it. A willingness to consider your hearing loss a fact of life will create a solid bridge to healing. This is the foundation upon which all hearing problems can find resolution.

There are two common philosophies people seem to adopt once hearing loss becomes a part of their lives: cover up the fact that you have it or tell others when the occasion is appropriate that you don't hear well. There are many variations between both themes but if you look at yourself honestly, you'll recognize where you stand in your own thinking.

The emotions a person feels when hearing loss is confirmed incorporates the full range of human experiences. Some are relieved that at last they know that this is the cause of their problem, that they're not losing their mind, and are grateful at the diagnosis. At the other extreme, some are horrified. It seems an unbelievable possibility that the problem could be wholly theirs. "Surely most people mumble!" they conclude.

So many of us react in so many different ways that predicting how you might experience hearing loss is quite a complex matter. Furthermore, your reactions to hearing loss do not necessarily correlate to the degree of impairment; that is, you can have a mild loss of hearing which impacts your life more profoundly than someone with more significant hearing loss. Your reactions will be most influenced by how you feel about yourself and the world around you, your personality type, and how other people close to you deal with your problem. The most important ground rule to bear in mind when looking at your issues as we progress through this chapter is, *you must be honest with yourself.*

Self Inquiry

If you're willing to be introspective about your hearing problem and consider solutions, this is the place to begin. Problems usually have at least two solutions that bring about healing: (1) change the situation, or (2) change how you feel, interact or react. The problem with *changing the situation* (if you're an unaided person with hearing loss) is that you could find yourself continually changing your environment and still not hearing well. You may also try to change the environment to avoid an unpleasant experience but it doesn't necessarily help you hear better.

On the other hand, the problem with *changing how you feel* is that it's an imposing challenge. It's very difficult to transform anger into love, frustration into understanding, or embarrassment into delight. Surely, it would seem that it doesn't happen quickly if at all. Nonetheless, it can happen. When people open themselves up to accepting hearing loss, change can occur very quickly. It's the most predictable criterion on which hearing aids will be found acceptable; perhaps even the only criterion. Changing how you feel about hearing loss and hearing aids also becomes apparent to people in your life, and by mere acceptance, relationships transform.

The definition of "change" is "giving up something for something else." The difficulty for anyone in making changes is that it requires giving up something to which they've grown accustomed. It feels less certain, and sometimes frighteningly unfamiliar. Most of us find we're not skilled in making changes. It's usually something we find uncomfortable. Even good changes are known to cause stress. A move to a better house, getting a higher paying job, or even winning the lottery cause high stress. We tend to want to stick to "the familiar." Yet, going from dysfunction to adjustment necessitates change. To avoid stress, most of us unknowingly tend to stick to bad situations. I've often thought that there should be a course teaching students during their last year of high school how to gracefully make changes in their lives. How better adjusted to life's experiences we'd all be.

Perception has everything to do with the degree of adjustment, acceptance and solutions you embrace with regard to your hearing loss. Many people with hearing loss report they have altered their view of the world around them in an unhealthy way. People who were once soft spoken and gentle sometimes become outspoken and annoyed; others who were once alive with spirit and energy may grow pensive and withdrawn. Those close to them notice these changes and are saddened by it. If you aren't aware of such changes, if in fact they exist, it could be because they usually develop slowly over a period of years.

If you have the courage to really look at the impact hearing loss has had in your life, the following exercise may prove to be revealing. When completed, read the same list to someone who knows you well (your spouse, a grown child or a close friend) and ask this person to respond *how he or she believes you operate in the world.*

Exercise #1

If the statements feel mostly accurate write True; if they feel mostly inaccurate, write False:

1)_____ I don't hear well because other people mumble, don't enunciate clearly enough, or talk too softly for me to hear.

2)_____ Since I've had this hearing loss, I can't do all the things I'd like to do.

3)_____ People don't dare make jokes about my hearing trouble in my presence.

4)_____ I don't mingle with as many people (old and/or new acquaintances) as I used to because I don't hear well.

5)_____ I just can't be seen wearing a hearing aid.

6)_____ If I'm left alone in a conversation, I don't understand or trust what I hear.

7)_____ I know people think I'm not as sharp as I used to be because I don't hear as well as I once did.

8)_____ If I don't want to hear what someone says the first time, I'll remain quiet; it's a waste of my time trying to hear when I can't.

9)_____ I just can't seem to assert myself the way I used to (or as others do) since I lost my ability to hear well.

10)_____ It's difficult for me to accept I actually have a hearing loss.

11)____ I know I'm the source of the problem because of my hearing loss; when I miss what somebody says, it's not their fault.

12)____ Even though I have a hearing loss, I still do all the things I used to do.

13)____ I have humorous things happen to me as a result of my not hearing well.

14)____ In spite of my hearing loss, I'm careful not to give up any relationships I have in my life, or lose out on any potential relationships, by staying home too much.

15)____ I would not think of hiding the fact that I was wearing a hearing aid.

16)____ I feel completely at ease communicating with anyone in most environments even though I have hearing loss.

17)____ Despite my hearing loss, other people do not think less of me than before my loss developed.

18)____ I don't mind asking people to repeat what was said if I didn't hear it.

19)____ As my hearing loss has developed, I have made a systematic effort to compensate for it by being more outgoing.

20)____ It's easy for me to think of myself as having a hearing loss.

<u>Note</u>: Before you read the following interpretation which will give away the design of this exercise, be sure you and your partner complete it fully.

Interpretation

Statements 1 through 10 are the reverse of 11 through 20, respectively. For example, statement 3 is opposite to statement 13. There are two built-in veracity checks: one is that however you responded to a particular statement, if you're honest with yourself, you should have responded opposite to its corresponding statement. The other check is the way in which your partner responded.

Did you respond consistently to both sides of the statements, True on one, False on the other? Did your partner agree with you? If not, you may want to look carefully at the content of those statements. Are you procrastinating? Do you spend a lot of time with negative thinking about your hearing loss? Are you blaming others?

Or is your outlook healthy? Do you tend to think more positively in handling your hearing loss? Do you try and find the lighter side? Are you just as engaged in life as before you developed loss of hearing?

Once you've examined the way you and your par
the same statements, you may well find that you
who has prevented finding your own solutions. Thi.
an attempt to change who you are, but rather, to *change a.*
how you interact in the world.

Denying Hearing Loss

If your hearing healthcare provider informs you that you have an irreversible sensorineural hearing loss, despite the fact that more than 34 million other Americans share the same challenge, this is not welcomed news. However, it's quite another story if you don't believe it or choose to do nothing about it.

Most standard dictionaries define *denial* as *the refusal to believe* or *the act of disowning.* It's rejection of the notion that your hearing is an issue. This being so, you not only disown the condition, you decline help because logic dictates that you cannot seek help for something that does not exist. Although true denial of hearing loss is rare, resisting help is common. The following kinds of refrains are ones you yourself may made:

- "Nobody hears everything!"
- "Don't talk to me from another room and I'll hear great!"
- "It doesn't bother me!"
- "I just ask people to speak up!"
- "Only my wife (or husband) complains about it!"
- "I ignore it!"

Often, early resistance provides a useful function by allowing people time to recover from the initial shock of knowing they have a hearing loss. But some trap themselves here for years. To resist the notion of hearing loss implies you hear well, and this resistance is really self-deception.

Mechanisms of resistance can become an integral part of the way people operate in the world. The more sophisticated and highly developed their compensatory responses, the easier it may be to deny the problem. For example, some may have others help them hear, like asking others to repeat, rephrase, speak up and so forth. Without realizing it, they may grow skilled at favoring an ear, tuning one person in and another out, repeating what they think they hear to confirm its accuracy, reducing background noises, making educated guesses, watching facial movements and expressions as l as gestures and body language. These are all excellent and cessary ways to hear and understand better, but as suggested earlier, the irony is people can get stuck believing all of this will solve their problem, and it doesn't.

If you're wondering if you're experiencing resistance to hearing loss as you read this book, go back to the previous exercise to know. If you were in true denial, you probably wouldn't have picked up this book (although you could read it and say, "That's not me they're talking about!"). If you're well aware of your own hearing loss, but deny its presence when others inquire, that's not denial, it's conceal- ment. So, congratulations! At least you're willing to look at the problem. This is where we must begin.

It's been said that uncorrected hearing loss is more noticeable than hearing aids because the act of concealing a hearing loss is doomed to fail. It can make a person appear foolish, inattentive, disinterested, confused, senile or cognitively impaired. A person operating at this level needs to understand the serious emotional hardships imposed on oneself, the spouse, family and friends. Denying, resisting or minimizing the impact the loss has in one's life (or in the life of others) does not solve the problem. Having others "hear" for you is not the answer either. In fact, these things compound the problem in close relationships. "Why should I carry the burden?" an honest but resentful spouse will ask!

You might feel annoyed that you have a hearing loss but your spouse is annoyed that you do nothing about it. You may isolate yourself from family gatherings because you can't hear, feel foolish or embarrassed, but your family feels abandoned and dismissed that they aren't important enough to you when you isolate yourself from them. If you're a person unwilling to seek help, it can even create the feeling in loved ones and friends that you're quite selfish or irresponsible.

Co-Dependent Behavior

In 2005,[1] I published a study that explored who audiologists felt were more resistant to hearing aids, men or women. Over half of the practitioners surveyed (about 54 percent) reported they felt men were more resistant; about 34 percent felt it was equal; and only 9 percent of respondents reported women as being more resistant. If you're a man resisting the notion of hearing aids, so long as family members continue to serve your endless listening and hearing needs by repeating what you miss, interpreting messages, allowing you to avoid the telephone, without the need for you to seek professional help to solve this problem, you're in a co-dependent relationship. In fact, your spouse may have become so good at this behavior that it fools you into believing you actually hear adequately! That is, she has essentially become your ears. In some relationships this may be cut short once the hearing loss progresses. In other relationships as hearing loss gets worse, the spouse is Johnny-on-the-Spot and feels an increased demand on her to help you, digging an ever deeper trench of co-dependence. Either way, it is co-dependence, and it's not healthy. More than anything, it deprives you of your <u>hearing independence</u> which translates to social isolation, the very thing we need to prevent as we get older because aging usually creates more isolation than we want. To compound it by untreated hearing loss is nothing short of a shame.

In my patients willing to give up this co-dependency, I've seen a rebirth of marriages, newfound love and warmth among family members (especially children so frustrated and angry at your unwillingness to get help), and greater work efficiency. Regarding the latter, I fit hearing aids on a few psychiatrists in my career who had finally reached the end, unable to hear their patients correctly. Hearing aids changed their lives.

Isolationism

The personal tragedy of untreated hearing loss is the isolation that results from avoiding all the situations that make hearing a challenge. These also happen to be the situations that have made life so enjoyable. These include going to plays, movies, maybe giving up a favorite restaurant because it's too noisy, even giving up a certain relationship or two because someone speaks too softly.

Ultimately what this can lead to is the sense that you live in your own world. Once you've broken away from the "outside world," your reality is made up of two rather distinct and separate worlds: yours and the outside world. The longer you remain separate from this outside world, the more alienated you can feel about it, the more fear you can sense about having to deal with it at all on any basis, simply because it's no longer comfortable, and it's no longer safe. The natural progression of this is giving up more and more pleasures in life in order to operate your life within your own comfort zone. The easy resolve is to face the need to solve this self-imposed "exile" from the world by seeing if hearing aids are the answer. This is an enormous bridge to cross for many people, but it is the bridge to healing.

Procrastination

Making the decision to try hearing aids is not an easy one for some people, especially if sometimes you hear beautifully, and other times poorly. Loved ones may also observe this to be true. This gives the false impression that you have a *listening issue*, not a *hearing problem*. This is the elusive nature of hearing loss because it's frequency-sensitive. That is, you may hear your father perfectly, but cannot hear a co-worker. You may believe room acoustics are the problem, or that it's other people—they talk like they have marbles in their mouth or "mumble." You may hear people differently because some voices project better than others. Men are usually easier to hear than women or children for those with high frequency hearing loss. And the environment plays a significant role, especially around noise. The bottom line is that the configuration of loss you have may allow you to hear some voices well, others poorly.

Putting off the hearing evaluation (or hearing aids) can be based on what seems like valid logic:

- "I'm too young!"
- "It's not bad enough yet!"
- "No one I know likes their hearing aids!"
- "We just can't afford it now!"
- "After we paint the house!"
- "Tom has a hearing loss and doesn't wear hearing aids and he gets along just fine!" (but of course Tom really doesn't).

Such people recognize their hearing loss but try to find every excuse not to do anything about it. This is procrastination. Hearing problems may be minimized in order to justify not pursuing treatment. And in the presence of other health concerns, this may seem like just one more issue on the list:

- "After I do my teeth!"
- "I don't want to spend my children's inheritance!"
- "If only Medicare paid for it!"
- "Maybe after that trip to Hawaii" (or that new car)

Any of this sound familiar? If so, we'll explore this more thoroughly. Fasten your seatbelt.

Emotions Behind Hearing Loss

How you deal with hearing loss probably parallels how you deal with life. We all develop patterns by three to five years of age which become programmed into our personality. While you may wish to act and react differently, to a certain extent, it means deprogramming (and reprogramming) yourself. Despite such imposing challenges against change, to attempt change precludes the *desire* or *intent* to change. As you are about to discover, failure to change by not seeking help for your hearing loss is linked to a myriad of emotional issues, some permanent, but most preventable.

I encourage anyone willing to explore their internal emotional processes to consider consulting a psychotherapist (individually or as a couple). Such an unbiased personal sounding board so often proves to be a very rewarding, productive and nurturing experience.

Let's explore some of the emotions we commonly see in people with untreated hearing loss.

Avoidance, Anxiety & Social Phobias

As presented earlier, aging often correlates to isolation because with progressing years we lose friends and relatives, it becomes more difficult to get out, we have less energy, and so forth. Thus, we can find ourselves more isolated. Untreated hearing loss compounds the matter. The experience of separation from others is not limited to the over-fifty crowd. I've seen many patients in their twenties and thirties give up their favorite activities because of their inability to hear adequately. I've seen high school students refuse to wear hearing aids because they feared peer ridicule. They sadly preferred to be left alone and miss out on social interaction rather than risk being seen wearing hearing aids. [Since the advent of open ear hearing aids in 2003, this situation has done a one-eighty.]

Social phobias can and do commonly develop from untreated hearing loss.[2] A social phobia is a form of anxiety; a persistent fear of social or performance situations in which embarrassment may occur. For example, if you avoided a particular social obligation with your significant other because you feared the embarrassing conse-quences of your hearing loss, and these situations were persistent, excessive and recurrent for more than six months, you probably have a social phobia.

If you have noticed that you've been avoiding social situations as described, you should be concerned. Fundamentally, you're cutting yourself off from the nurturing people who make you feel loved in the world. Clearly not a healthy choice. Apart from hearing loss, anxiety disorders are serious medical conditions affecting more than 19 million American adults and can grow progressively worse if untreated. Through the 1990s, anxiety disorders in the U.S. grew by more than 50 percent and pose a major public health concern. Interestingly, according to the National Institute on Deafness and Other Communication Disorders (NIDCD), hearing loss is the third most prevalent chronic condition in older Americans. So, if you're an older American experiencing hearing loss, you have much greater risk for isolation and avoidance of common pleasures in life—not to mention depression.

Depression

More than 22 percent of Americans ages 18 and older suffer from a diagnosable mental disorder in a given year,[3] and major depressive disorder is the leading cause of disability in the U.S. and established market economies worldwide.[4] Onset of depression usually occurs in the twenties, impacting twice as many women as men. Unfortunately, for those with hearing loss, the likelihood of also suffering from depression is increased.[5]

Although these are staggering statistics, it's important to understand that depression is not a natural part of aging. It can be prevented and is treatable in about 80 percent of older adults. A major source of depression, especially in older adults, stems from untreated hearing loss. The simple action of wearing hearing aids can resolve the associated depression. In older adults, this should be pursued aggressively, since depression is also commonly associated with anxiety and other ailments. As we age, our normal coping abilities diminish. It's so important to restore as much normal functioning as we can, at any age, but especially in these later years.

Often we think that what we feel inside remains hidden. It is easy to forget that those we love can usually see past this thin veil. And rest assured, if depression is there, and they love you, they'll eventually see it, and will be suffering along with you. In clinical terms, depression is often described as *anger turned inward*.

Anger

Anger is a kind of stepchild to depression. When left untreated, people with depression can be difficult to be around, but something you may be surprised to hear is that you have a right to be angry! It's your body. Hearing is a needed and vital sense. Its loss influences almost every aspect of socialization. Every time you ask people to repeat themselves, it's a quiet reminder of a problem that does not go away.

The problem with anger is that it typically finds an outward vent. Eventually, you can become resentful and angry at others over your own need to have things repeated. Worse yet, you may become angry when a family member suggests you should get help! You already know that, you just don't want to hear it from anyone. For some, this is just too painful.

The dynamics of this emotion are fairly simple. You become angry that you're not hearing. The family is upset that this "stubborn person" isn't doing more about the hearing loss. Some hard of hearing people, oblivious to the impact their hearing loss has on others, may ask to have things repeated in a blaming manner. This leads others to feel that the communication problem extends *to them,* and therefore your anger gets them angry!

If you recognize that anger is an issue, you may also discover that you are as angry (or disappointed) with the world as you are with yourself. This further locks you into the separation crisis between "your world" and the "outside world" discussed earlier. Perhaps you desperately want to make a change and escape from your world, but don't know how or where to turn. Seeking audiologic counsel is a first step. Indecision may keep you angry and upset. If you continue ignoring the problem, the issues surrounding it are further perpetuated. If you find solace in reverting to denial of the problem, it's a short-lived reprieve because you've already awakened to the truth of your situation.

For many people, unexpressed inner turmoil finally shifts from its simmering, hidden view, to boiling over. People around you are less likely to understand from where this hostility arises, especially if you yourself are not in touch with it. You risk relationships with friends and family disintegrating as fast as your quality of life.

If you are of an angry nature, and if it is hearing loss-related, hopefully you will become attuned to the fact that your upset originates from your failure to seek help. Thus, no one but you can really solve this dilemma. Through such enlightenment, you will also discover a renewed sense of calm because now you can take back control of your life.

Selfishness and Resentment

If we ever question how difficult it is to live with another person, all we have to do is look at the divorce rate. Health issues aside, it's not easy. Now throw into the mix a partner who refuses to get help for a health problem, regardless of the condition, now you have a problem. If this problem is untreated hearing loss, a common reaction of a partner is anger or disappointment that their loved one will do nothing about the problem. This then, in very subtle ways, begins to characterize you as a person.

Coming to terms with hearing loss can be a very slow journey for many. If you expect others to compensate for your loss of hearing instead of assuming this responsibility yourself, you will likely set up a fertile environment for strained family relationships. Your negligence may rightfully be seen as a selfish act. Of course you're entitled to expect others not to speak to you from another room, or in the presence of such cacophony as a loud television, a vacuum cleaner or music. But in the absence of wearing hearing aids, the family shouldn't be expected to manipulate the household for your convenience, especially when it's at the expense of others you care about.

If you're out socially without hearing aids, you already know how frustrated your friends and loved ones are over seeing you miss out on conversation. If you're in a movie theater (if in fact you're not avoiding theaters altogether) and your spouse or friend must continuously repeat the onscreen dialogue, you might be hearing a lot of, "Shhh!" from those seated near you. In the meantime, you, your partner and maybe others around you have just missed another line of dialogue.

Eventually, for most every relationship, all the rigmarole required by loved ones to accommodate your hearing problem at the expense of their untold inconveniences will lead to resentment. Why has your problem suddenly become their problem? Why is it their responsibility to be your ears? Why should they be solving your hearing problems?

Frustration and Defeat

I've already presented frustration as a common experience for everyone surrounding untreated hearing loss. When you look at such family dynamics, frustration touches about everyone. It's very easy for family members to forget that you do not hear well. After all, there's no melon-size growth on the top of your head to remind them, no bandages, no walker. Because you give the general appearance of looking so normal, others may expect you to *hear normally*. Your kids or spouse may continue to talk to you from other rooms, or with a back turned or with a pencil in the mouth. Inadvertently, your loved ones are aiding and abetting without realizing it.

Worse, you tell your physician that you believe you have some hearing loss and are surprised what you're told. Research has shown that, first, your physician will not test you nor will he or she likely refer you to a hearing healthcare professional. To add insult to injury, you're probably told: "Don't worry about it. Everyone gets a little hearing loss eventually. I have a little myself but I just ignore it!" If your physician has told you ignore it, it may perhaps be well-intended, but it's downright incorrect and misguided information that will merely add to your mounting frustrations. You should know you're not alone. In 2004, I reported that 86 percent of physicians in the U.S. *did not* screen for hearing loss. In five years since, this trend has moved in the wrong direction—to 87 percent.[6]

During the initial stages of hearing loss you may have actually laughed at many misunderstood words. I was with my wife at the hardware store when I thought she said, "Do you need some *coffee?*"

I took the comment personally because I incorrectly assumed she thought I was not paying attention, but she had said, "Do you need some *caulking!*"

One time when we were about to get dressed for a party, I asked my wife what I should wear. She turned to me and as clear as a bell said, "Leave your clothes!" Leave my clothes? Hardly, I thought! I only heard it correctly when she repeated it. "*Leisure* clothes!" Good thing she repeated it!

I've also experienced hearing everything seemingly quite clearly but none of it making sense. And I have normal hearing! Repeating doesn't help because with a hearing loss at specific frequencies, the same words are expressed at the same frequencies where you don't hear well.

The humor of mistakes seems to eventually dwindle. What remains are the day-to-day frustrations. This can culminate into mixed emotions as we've discussed, especially annoyance and anger fueled by frustrations. A frequently heard comment by the person with hearing loss, as well as the family is, "I can't stand it anymore!" In fact, the longer untreated hearing loss persists, the greater the frustrations <u>for everyone</u>.

When frustration upon frustration over years occurs, there's a real sense of defeat by everyone in the family, including you. You make every effort to hear. You listen, you struggle, you're attentive, you make every effort to connect to this outside world, but it entails so much frustration and defeat that it becomes easier to withdraw. In almost every other health problem, you'd have received treatment. You wouldn't have put yourself and your loved ones through these hoops. To do nothing is resignation, concession, submission and surrender. It does nothing to lessen the burden on anyone. Such inaction is actually self-defeating, and shouldn't even be an option. (If you already wear hearing aids and feel defeated, explore all other choices available to you, *many included in this book*.)

Embarrassment

Probably the single most common experience among people with untreated hearing loss (and their family) is embarrassment. Second-guessing what you think you hear, offering inappropriate responses, missing the punch line to a joke, or getting wrong directions are small examples of what you and loved ones experience. Struggling to hear can put others ill at ease.

Much research indicates that sufferers do not pursue help for themselves because the thought of wearing hearing aids is embarrassing. Ironically, failure to get help usually proves to be more embarrassing. With the open ear hearing aid fittings of recent years, this trend has shifted. The cosmetic appeal of these exceptionally inconspicuous hearing aids has attracted wearers who would never have considered amplification on any other basis. As a result, embarrassment about hearing aid use has significantly been reduced in many cases, even eliminated. In the hearing healthcare world of today, hearing aids and other appropriate amplification accessories offer anyone with loss of hearing the most efficient avenue to independent hearing. These devices allow you to break free of your dependence on others, and can make all the difference in strengthening your relationship with those around you rather than fueling embarrassment and other ill feelings by ignoring the problem.

Rejection

Bill was a likeable but boisterous man. He told funny jokes but he told them with such volume that strangers thirty feet away laughed.

He was a source of constant entertainment as well as embarrassment to his wife and friends. Sitting in a restaurant, he'd talk about people's personal problems. It wasn't that his friends didn't want their problems discussed, they just didn't want the entire restaurant to hear about it. It was as if Bill had no sense of where he was or what was appropriate. No one suspected, until I met Bill, his wife and others for lunch one day, that he had a marked loss of hearing. Bill knew it, but he wasn't about to let anyone else in on his secret. His refusal for help cost him the relationships of people who once truly loved and cared about him. However, his friends simply could no longer tolerate the humiliations that went along with the friendship.

Many hard of hearing people are rejected by others who do not recognize their condition. When others remain uninformed about why you may behave or interact the way you do, they're forced to draw wrong conclusions that carry undesirable consequences. You don't have to be vulnerable to social rejection. You have to experience this only a few times to know how painful it is. People may whisper behind your back, "Has he become senile?" "Is he functioning okay?" "Does Bill know he constantly offers incorrect replies in conversation?"

The ultimate rejection is you rejecting the outside world, continuing to live isolated in your safe but narrow space of not hearing well.

Sensory Deprivation

Sensory deprivation research was popular in the 1950s and told us much about the human experience in the absence of stimulation. John Lilly, MD[7] authored a few pop culture books on this subject matter, as well as fascinating scientific papers. He was the creator of the "Lilly Tank," where you could float on Epson salts sealed inside a tank, had no body awareness, no light and no sound.

As auditory, visual and sensual input diminishes with less stimulation to corresponding neural centers in the brain, the brain is not happy. Lilly's students subjected to these experiments generally could not tolerate the absence of sensory stimulation longer than a few hours or a few days. Besides altered realities, other complaints included feelings of disorientation and inability to concentrate. You should know that people who suffer from hearing loss (which is auditory deprivation) also report *the same symptoms*.

Solitary confinement in prisons is sensory deprivation to the extreme. Over time, it has been shown to cause permanent problems, most profoundly, *intolerance to social interaction.* Obviously, this effect is counterproductive to a society that desires paroled inmates to be acclimated back into society. By no coincidence, symptoms found among many people with untreated hearing loss (auditory deprivation) also include *intolerance to social interaction.* This is the "your world," "their world" syndrome.

Much of reality (what little we understand of it) is based on our very delicate sensory systems. Impairment to any one of our five senses *does result in an altered state of reality.* If you miss portions of communication and don't realize it, you're experiencing one thing while something else entirely may have been intended. When you experience auditory deprivation, your natural instinct is to avoid social situations because just like students in Lilly's experiments, not many people like living in an altered state of reality.

There's now reliable scientific evidence to document the fact that untreated hearing loss can lead to a variety of unhealthy emotional conditions. The Hearing Instrument Association in conjunction with the National Council on Aging ran a study with over 2,000 hard of hearing adults and over 1700 family members.[8] This study concluded that people who suffer from hearing loss were more likely to experience increased anger, frustration, paranoia, insecurity, instability, nervousness, tension, anxiety, irritability, discontentment, depression, being temperamental, fearful, more likely to be self-critical, suffer from a sense of inferiority, social phobias, be perceived as confused, disoriented or unable to concentrate. Experiencing only one of these would seem enough to inspire one to seek help, but unfortunately, many people with hearing loss tend to experience a variety of these unhealthy emotional states.

Furthermore, research shows that failure to stimulate hearing (the auditory portion of the brain) by not wearing hearing aids may result in a more rapid decline in speech recognition.[9-10] These reports were based on a substantial number of subjects who possessed at least a moderate degree of hearing loss in both ears but received only one hearing aid. As a result of auditory deprivation in the unaided ear, a reduction in speech recognition occurred. For some, when hearing loss is not addressed as a major health issue, the risks of negative emotional impact are high. These are consequences that can be avoided, but often are not because people don't realize the impact of untreated hearing loss. Now let's examine this impact.

Your Spouse or Significant Other

Probably the average person with hearing loss has experienced impatience at times causing them to be harsher on loved ones than they'd like, or insensitive, unkind or unfair. Once you've recognized your actions, you may feel guilty. You may wish you could have handled the situation differently but you just couldn't control yourself. More so, you may feel like it's a vicious cycle—you expect loved ones to be your ears, yet, those around you get fed up doing the hearing for you. It really is lose-lose.

I always include the spouse in conversations because they are the richest source of information. When I ask for their assessment, the common response is, "I'm so tired of repeating myself!" What you must understand is that everyone feels the same way. Though you may live in your own world, the problems are projected out into the world of those who hear.

Sadly, only 20 percent of people who suffer from hearing loss seek treatment through hearing aids. This speaks volumes about what spouses endure. It does not only mean louder television, repeating yourself throughout the day, and filling in parts of important conversations, it dangerously raises the level of anxiety in a healthy spouse married to someone with hearing loss. Your spouse will develop her or his own anxiety around your issues, which can start with annoyance and lead to anger, intolerance, a sense of hopelessness, and can even lead to depression. In some cases, I've seen my patients divorce. Struggling to communicate under these circumstances is exhausting.

Many people with untreated hearing loss feel they're not ready for hearing aids. Inspiring you to seek this needed help may be the most challenging task your spouse and family face. Change of course begins with your readiness. The rewards can dramatically improve lives and usually transforms relationships.

Expectations versus Actual Performance

If you're a person living in a non-amplified world, you no doubt have expectations about hearing that may not align with your performance. I've had family members with hearing loss refuse to get hearing aids, then go into situations expecting to hear. At the end of the evening, I'd point out how much conversation was missed.

People who haven't yet come to terms with their loss of hearing, or who have not fully admitted it to themselves, mistakenly believe that *they hear all they need to hear.* The truth is, *you only hear what your hearing capacity permits.* The illusion to oneself is two-fold: you not only fail to get important information but you don't even know it. The illusion to others is that they believe communication has occurred when in fact it hasn't. Thus, we not only have miscommunication, but multiple altered realties.

Exercise #2

Here's a little exercise that can help you better understand hearing loss. Divide the top of a blank sheet of paper into three sections: on the left, title it "Situations;" in the middle "Expectations;" and on the right, "Actual Performance."

List three to five situations or environments where you expect to hear regardless of whether or not you actually can. Your task is to rate the items under the "Expectations" and "Actual Performance" columns by selecting one of the following ratings:

NEVER - RARELY - SOMETIMES - OFTEN - ALWAYS

After you've completed this, take another piece of paper and list the same situations. Then have your partner or someone close to you complete how they think your expectations versus actual performance pan out. This makes for healthy discussion, and a great opportunity to compare and contrast perceptions. The more truthful you are with yourself, the more you'll gain from these insights.

Interpretation

If you've rated everything in the exercise the same for all situations, either you're an amazingly well adjusted person with hearing loss, or you're kidding yourself. It's unlikely that all hearing situations on your list will be evaluated equally even if you're well adjusted.

So, take a closer look at your list. Bear in mind that people with normal hearing will rate the situations of expectations and performance differently because of their varying listening environments. The difference indicates the magnitude of the problem; the greater the difference, the greater the problem. For many people with loss of hearing, it's typical to have expectations higher than performance levels. As a result, reactions to environmental situations that prove difficult can lead to the emotions we've discussed.

Acceptance and Moving On

Are you ready to make a positive change in your life? Do you want better communication? Do you want to do more to help yourself? Is the quality of your life important enough to you to make positive changes? Do you care enough about loved ones to make these changes? Can you accept that the "outside world" is safe enough for you to coexist?

You already recognize the trials and tribulations of insufficient hearing. Acceptance of hearing loss allows you to move on. It's that easy. You know that despite all your efforts, all your loved ones' efforts to compensate for you not hearing, nothing has gotten you through. This realization is essential before you can move on with clear vision. Coming to terms with the emotions surrounding your hearing builds your bridge to healing. Acceptance of your hearing loss allows you safe passage into the outside world.

References

1. Carmen R. (2005) Who are more resistant to hearing aid purchases—women or men? *Audiology Today* 17(2).
2. Carmen R and Uram S. (2002) Hearing loss and anxiety in adults. *The Hearing Journal* 55(4).
3. Reiger DA, Narrow WE, Rae DS, et al. (1993) The de facto mental and addictive disorders service system. Epidemiologic Catchment Area prospective 1-year prevalence rates of disorders and services. *Archives of General Psychiatry* 50(2):85-94.
4. Klerman GL, Weissman MM. (1989) Increasing rates of depression. *JAMA* 261(15):2229-35.
5. Bridges JA, Bentler RA. (1998) Relating hearing aid use to well-being among older adults. *The Hearing Journal* 51(7):39-44.
6. Kochkin, S. (July 2005) MarkeTrak VII: Hearing loss population tops 31 million people, *The Hearing Review* 12(7):16-29.
7. Lilly J. (1972) *The Center of the Cyclone: An Autobiography of Inner Space.* New York: Bantam Books.
8. Kochkin S and Rogin CM. (2000) Quantifying the obvious: the impact of hearing instruments on quality of life. *The Hearing Review* 7(1).
9. Silman S, et al. (1984) Late on-set auditory deprivation: effects of monaural versus binaural hearing aids. *J. Acoust. Soc. Am.* 76:1357-62.
10. Silman S, et al. (1992) Adult-onset auditory deprivation. *J. Am. Acad. Audiol.* 3:390-96.

Suggested Reading

Burkey, JM. (2006) *Baby Boomers and Hearing Loss: A Guide to Prevention and Care.* Chaphill, NC: Rutgers University Press.

Carmen, R. (2005) *How Hearing Loss Impacts Relationships: Motivating Your Loved One.* Sedona, AZ: Auricle Ink Publishers.

Harvey, MA. (2004) *Odyssey of Hearing Loss: Tales of Triumph.* San Diego, CA: Dawnsign Press.

Morris, RA. (2007) *On the Job with Hearing Loss.* New York: Morgan-James.

Myers, D.G. (2000) *A Quiet World.* New Haven, CT: Yale University Press.

CHAPTER TWO

Why Some Consumers Reject Hearing Aids But How You Could Love Them!

Sergei Kochkin, Ph.D.

Dr. Kochkin is Executive Director of the Better Hearing Institute (Washington, DC). He has 25 years of corporate experience as a market researcher and industrial psychologist. He has published close to 70 papers on the hearing loss population and the hearing aid market and conducted extensive customer satisfaction research on more than 30,000 hearing aid owners. He holds a Doctorate in psychology, an MBA in marketing, a Master's of Science in counseling and guidance, and a BA in physical anthropology and archaeology. Dr. Kochkin also maintains an interest in ancient cultures, comparative religion, meditation, and golf.

Recent research in the United States indicates that close to 32 million people have a hearing loss—nearly one in ten Americans. In addition, about 1.4 million school-age children have a hearing loss. The early identification and treatment of hearing loss in children are particularly critical because normal development of speech and language depend on hearing. It's important that you understand the prevalence of hearing loss and the fact that it cuts across all age groups. In fact, most people are amazed when they learn that 65 percent of people with hearing loss are below retirement age.[1] In focus groups with people who have rejected hearing aids, some people with hearing loss expressed the erroneous conclusions that they are rare or obscure individuals, "since so few people have hearing loss" or that their hearing loss "is a sign of aging." When shown that they were not alone and that most people with hearing loss are younger than they were, they tended to be more accepting of their hearing loss and therefore more willing to seek a hearing aid solution.

Conversations with experts in other countries generally recognize that close to ten percent of the populations in developed countries have problems with their hearing. I happen to believe the actual figure may be higher, because most studies have not included hearing loss populations in institutional settings such as nursing or retirement homes, the military, and prisons. Among the elderly, hearing loss is the third most serious health issue, following arthritis and hypertension.

The vast majority (close to 90-95 of people with hearing loss) can be helped by hearing aids. Because of major breakthroughs in hearing aid technology in recent years, we can now do a better job of matching technology with a candidate's lifestyle and communication needs. Yet, some purchased hearing aids still end up in their owners' drawers, unworn.[2] The good news is that many of the problems with hearing aids have been solved, and wearers can now expect improved communication with hearing aids as the rule, not the exception.

Why do some individuals have difficulty adjusting to hearing aids while others are doing so well that people around them don't even notice they're wearing them? What's different about successful hearing aid wearers? And why do only one in five individuals with hearing loss use hearing aids despite the proven value of amplification? Some interesting facts now coming to light may answer these questions.

Why Some People Reject Hearing Aids

More than 24 million people in the United States with hearing loss have never tried hearing aids as a solution. One research investigation polled close to 3,000 individuals with self-reported hearing loss regarding their reluctance to try hearing aids.[3] Here are some of the reasons why consumers have declined to pursue them.

1. Inadequate Information

Many people are not aware they have a significant hearing loss and therefore are in need of information that would help them recognize it. Most people lose hearing gradually. In most cases, it's slowly progressive. During this time, both the person with hearing loss and family members adapt to it, often not even realizing that they're doing this. The number one reason why people buy their very first hearing aid is the "recognition that their hearing got worse;" usually this means they made embarrassing mistakes in society due to their untreated hearing loss. Thus, one of the first things individuals with suspected hearing loss should do is determine if they exhibit some of the signs of hearing loss.

2. Stigma and Cosmetics

Some people reject hearing aids because they're concerned with the stigma of hearing loss or are in a state of denial, and thus they try to hide it from others. It's unfortunate, but many people, because they have less than perfect hearing, believe they are inferior, unintelligent, or simply less lovable. They believe other people will think they're getting older or will view them as less competent, less attractive, and so on. They may have shame regarding their hearing loss. This is partly due to the fact that we live in a youth-oriented, airbrushed society that stresses physical perfection as an important human attribute.

As you previously read in this book, cosmetics no longer need to be a barrier to obtaining amplification. Since the 1990s, technological advances have permitted the hearing aid industry to develop hearing instruments like completely-in-the-canal (CIC) hearing aids or the new open fit, which are virtually invisible (see Chapter 3, Figure 3-1). In fact, research shows that 90 percent of consumers perceived these hearing aids to be completely invisible. Based on your hearing needs and the physical characteristics of your ears, you might be a candidate for these "invisible devices." If you're not, rest assured that in-the-canal (ITC) devices, although larger, are available to fit many hearing losses and are not terribly noticeable.

Understand though, that once you begin hearing through amplifcation and once it has enhanced your quality of life, cosmetics will be of lesser concern to you. Research shows that people who have come to enjoy their hearing aids rate even the largest hearing aids as cosmetically appealing as compared to some of the smaller, in-the-ear models.[4] Some hearing instruments even come in bright colors—dispelling the myth that they're something to be ashamed of or hide! So, stigma and cosmetic concerns of the past five years are now substantially diminished, and for most who put these on their ears, completely resolved.

3. Misdirected Medical Guidance

Many people have received misinformation from well-intending physicians about their hearing loss and the extent to which it can be helped. For instance, many physicians have advised their patients that they're not candidates for hearing aids if they have hearing loss in one ear and good hearing in the other (unilateral hearing loss); if they have "nerve deafness" (an obsolete term for sensorineural hearing loss); or if the hearing loss still allows them to conduct a conversation in quiet. Many times, the doctor's opinion will derive from the fact that the patient and doctor are able to conduct a face-to-face conversation in the secluded and usually quiet exam room.

Much of this unintentional misinformation comes from family physicians who don't specialize in hearing problems. In fact, most physicians (except ear, nose, and throat specialists) receive very little training in medical school in the areas of hearing loss and hearing aids. The only helpful information will come from those who specialize in hearing loss.

4. Not Realizing the Importance of Hearing

Another reason for rejection of hearing aids is that people have forgotten how important hearing is to their quality of life. We live in such a visually oriented society that often hearing plays a secondary role. As you know from your own experience or from this book, people who cannot hear well often have lives filled with anxiety, insecurity, isolation, and depression. People gradually withdraw from family and friends because without auditory contact they lose the feeling of being connected. In essence, they grow numb to the world around them. But in the real world (or as Dr. Carmen suggested, "the outside world,") interpersonal communication is critical.

5. Erroneous Belief that Hearing Aids Don't Work

A significant number of people with hearing loss mistakenly believe that hearing aids are not effective for what they're designed to do. Many people judge hearing aids based on what they've seen their grandparents wear—a large, clunky box about the size of a pack of cigarettes with wires coming out of it.

Recent research with consumers utilizing a variety of hearing aids (high technology as well as older technology aids 1-5 years old) indicated that 90 percent of hearing aid wearers reported satisfaction (defined as *somewhat satisfied, satisfied,* or *very satisfied)* with the ability of the hearing aids to improve their hearing, and 93 percent reported that hearing aids have improved the quality of their life.[4] If this research had been conducted twenty years ago, this high satisfaction factor probably would not have been even 35 percent. A significant number of people reported satisfaction with their hearing aids in quiet situations (90 percent) as well as in very difficult situations such as restaurants (74 percent), places of worship (74 percent), or large groups (63 percent).

In research with more than 30,000 consumers, I've learned that not everyone benefits equally in all listening situations, nor do all types of hearing aid circuitry perform the same in difficult listening situations. For example, the average hearing aid achieves a 51 percent satisfaction rating in noisy situations; yet some technologies, notably programmable hearing aids with multiple microphones (known as *directional* hearing aids), have achieved satisfaction ratings as high as 90 percent.[5] While few practitioners dispense these analog programmable hearing aids any longer on which the study was based, what's relevant is that all digital hearing aids are programmable.

Also, only about 69 percent of consumers are satisfied with hearing aids on the telephone, yet some instruments, such as completely-in-the-canal (CIC) hearing aids, perform better on the phone as well as outdoors because they're located just inside the entrance of the ear canal and produce less feedback while on the phone. Much of this satisfaction may also be due to diminished wind noises outdoors, a sense of more natural amplification, and the need for somewhat less power, resulting in increased tolerance of background noise. Understand that hearing aids in the "Telephone" position (T-coil) completely eliminate feedback (see Chapter 5).

In the last five years, smaller behind-the-ear open fit hearing aids have become the rage in America. They have solved some of the long-term complaints of consumers: the sound of their voice is more natural, and it no longer feels as if they're hearing in a barrel (occlusion); the fit is more comfortable because their hearing aid shell is not in their ear; it is in fact less visible than in the ear devices; there's less whistling and feedback; the sound quality is more natural; and wearers believe they're achieving more benefit.[6]

Since the digital revolution, now more than 90 percent of hearing aids sold in America are digital. Have digital hearing aids improved the consumer's experience? Our recent survey with 2,300 consumers of hearing aids associated the use of digital hearing instruments with significantly higher overall satisfaction and benefit; improved sound quality; reduction in feedback; improved performance in noisy situations; and greater utility in a number of important listening situations.[4] With continued advances in digital signal processing and the coming wireless revolution, I'm confident that the utility of hearing aids will improve dramatically in the next decade.

6. Failure to Trust in a Hearing Aid Dispensing Professional

Another key reason some people hold off their purchase is: "I do not trust hearing health providers who fit hearing aids!" Yet, the data show that 93 percent of consumers felt satisfied with their hearing aid dispensing professional.[4] It's certainly worth mentioning that the training, education, and experience of dispensers of hearing aids have greatly increased over the years, for both *audiologists* and *hearing instrument specialists* (see Appendix II for definitions).

7. Unrecognized Value of Hearing Aids

Many people who have avoided amplification tend to believe there's little value in hearing aids. They mistakenly assume that "hearing aids will not work for them" and therefore they will not derive any benefit. Both consumers and physicians have little knowledge of the potential benefit of hearing aids. Since the new millennium, large-scale research has examined the impact of hearing aids on quality of life for people who use hearing aids in the United States.[7] While I have devoted a full chapter to this research, it's important that we summarize this impact here.

In my humble opinion, I cannot think of a consumer product with such an impressive list of potential benefits: greater earning power; improved interpersonal relationships; reduced discrimination toward the person with the hearing loss; reduced difficulty in communicating; less need to compensate for hearing loss; reduced anger and frustration; reduction in depression and anxiety; enhanced emotional stability; reductions in paranoid feelings; reduced social phobias; greater belief that you are in control of your life; reduced self-criticism; increased self-esteem; improved perceptions of mental acuity; improved health status; greater level of outgoingness (e.g., extraversion); and greater likelihood of participating in groups. I challenge anyone to name a product or a service with this impressive list of benefits. When I presented these findings to a group of medical doctors, one prominent physician stated, "I was not aware of the seriousness of hearing loss and the potential for hearing aids to alleviate the problem. Every doctor in the world must be made aware of these findings!"

8. Feeling Priced Out of the Market

Some people with hearing loss simply do not have the disposable income that would enable them to afford today's modern hearing aids and healthcare treatment. Based on the known benefits of hearing aids improving quality of life, there's some effort being generated to see if more government programs such as Medicare will cover hearing aids.If the person with a hearing loss is a child, many local and state governments offer hearing aids at no or reduced cost. Check to see if you qualify for free aids or for a reduced price for hearing aids through your union, employer, the Veterans Administration, your insurance provider, your HMO, or your local Lions Club. There's also a current initiative to provide a $500 tax credit per hearing aid for children, Boomers, and seniors. To make your voice heard on this bill, visit www.hearingaidtaxcredit.org. Also we have listed charitable foundations that provide help with hearing aids at www.betterhearing.org under "Resources" (Financial).

Twelve Ways to Optimize Your Chances of Being a Satisfied Hearing Aid Wearer

There is nothing more important to the manufacturers of hearing aids and hearing healthcare professionals than your satisfaction with their product and services. Like other smart professionals, they know that satisfied clients lead to repeat business and to positive word-of-mouth advertising for their products. The hearing aid industry is interested in delighting you, in meeting your needs and exceeding your expectations. The people-oriented hearing aid industry fosters significant interaction and communication between the person with hearing loss and hearing health professionals to assure that they've done all things possible to meet your needs. You have a role to play in assuring your satisfaction with hearing aids. So, I would like to offer some suggestions for optimizing the chances that you'll be one of these delighted hearing aid wearers.

1. Meeting Your Needs

Simply stated, satisfaction is having your needs, desires, or expectations met. Another way of looking at satisfaction is feeling fulfilled; based on promises met by your hearing healthcare provider. You have very specific needs, and the purpose of the hearing healthcare provider is to find out what your needs are and how to meet them. Thus, during the process of rediscovering your hearing, it's important to determine what these needs are, what outcomes you're looking for, and most importantly, how you'll know when you've met your needs. The clearer you are about this, the more likely a positive outcome. Many people go to their hearing healthcare practitioner with a vague concept of their needs: "I can't hear," or "It seems as if people are mumbling more," or worse yet, "My wife says I don't listen to her."

I believe you will have a more fulfilling hearing aid experience if you dig deeper to comprehend the impact your hearing loss has had on your life emotionally, behaviorally, mentally, and socially. A number of chapters in this book can help you meet this challenge. Write the issues down because they will become a roadmap for both you and your hearing healthcare professional. Also, many hearing healthcare professionals have assessment scales that will help you understand problems caused by your hearing loss. Once you know your problems, you can better identify your expected outcomes. It's your personal needs list, and when it's fulfilled, it will bring a smile to your face and the faces of your loved ones. This list also becomes a contract between you and your hearing care professional.

2. Motivation

Advanced hearing aid technology can now compensate for most hearing losses, but millions of hearing aid candidates still are not ready to accept this fact. Is there a missing link? I think so. People with hearing loss are in different stages of readiness. At one extreme, the individual is in denial about the hearing loss. If either a family member or a professional insists on hearing aids at this point, behavior is unlikely to change, and most likely such a person would be dissatisfied if wearing hearing aids.

Individuals highly motivated to improve their hearing have an infinitely better chance of success with hearing aids. Such motivated people recognize their hearing loss and are open to change. They tend to seek out relevant information related to their hearing loss and the technology needed to alleviate the hearing problem. The most highly motivated hearing aid candidates have a willingness to discuss their feelings about their hearing problem and explore some hearing options that might be available to them. When fitted with hearing aids, they eagerly explore their new technology, discuss problems during follow-up visits with their hearing health professional, and patiently learn to adapt to their technology.

3. Positive Attitude

The most important personality trait that one could possess is a positive attitude, not just toward the process of obtaining hearing aids but toward life in general. This means a willingness to try hearing aids, adapt to new solutions, and keep frustration at a minimum when obstacles arise. If you view your circumstances as beyond your control, there's a higher probability that you'll be less successful in adapting to change, including hearing aid use.

Hearing aid studies have shown that people who have a positive outlook on life do better with hearing aids.[8] They have a positive self-image and believe they're in control of their life. My recommendation is take charge and be determined to improve the quality of your life with today's modern hearing aids.

4. Age of Your Hearing Aids

It's human nature to want to keep your hearing aids as long as possible in order to maximize value. However, hearing aids do wear out over time, ear canals change in shape, and the pattern of your hearing loss is likely to change in time. In the research that I've conducted, customer satisfaction was at its highest in the first year of use (78 percent). After five years of use, satisfaction dropped significantly to 58 percent, and after ten years of use even lower to 51 percent.[4]

So, it's important that you make sure that both the physical and audiological fit of your hearing aids is optimized for your hearing loss today rather than the way it was five, ten, or fifteen years ago. I would recommend that you replace your hearing aids every five years (if affordable) or when there have been significant advances in technology.

5. Choice of Technology

I've conducted extensive research across dozens of technologies. There is no doubt that customers are more satisfied with programmable, digital, and directional technology.[4,5] Advanced digital technology allows the hearing healthcare professional to adjust the hearing aid to your specific hearing loss characteristics with more precision. If the product does not meet your needs, then the hearing healthcare professional can adjust the hearing aid at the office versus sending it back to the manufacturer for adjustment.

With advancements in hearing aid technology has come a corresponding improvement in computer software that acoustically fits your hearing instruments to your specific needs. For example, some manufacturers store hundreds of "real world" sounds in the computer and allow you to see how your hearing aids will sound in those situations. This tremendous feature allows the hearing care practitioner to dynamically adjust the hearing aids based on your personal reaction to sounds.

A second advanced feature to consider is directional hearing aids. They have either two or three microphones in them. Because of their design, they're able to reduce some annoying background noise and improve your ability to understand speech in many difficult listening situations. Conducting three studies on directional hearing aids, I found a 17 percent customer satisfaction improvement in two studies and a 26 percent improvement in another.[5,9] The latter achieved a 90 percent customer satisfaction rating, the highest I have ever seen for a hearing aid. If you're an active person, then directional hearing aids could be suitable for you.

6. Controls on Your Hearing Aid

Your goal is to purchase a hearing aid that never needs adjustments. It should graciously determine the volume you need and adjust its directionality by sensing if you're in a quiet area or in a variety of noisy situations. A completely digital hearing aid, when it comes across steady state noise (like in an airplane cabin or around an air conditioner) should improve your hearing comfort in these situations by making the sounds more tolerable. In addition, it should not give you feedback as it amplifies sounds around you. It should restore your ability to enjoy some soft sounds (e.g., leaves rustling, bubbling of a fish tank, etc.) while sensing very loud sounds and making them comfortable for you (loud sounds should never be painful to your ears).

While the industry has in principle developed automatic hearing instruments, some people need to personally control them. Research has shown, especially among experienced wearers, that some people (roughly a third) still need either a volume control, multiple memory switch (quiet versus noisy situation switch), or a remote control in order to control volume or to access different hearing aid strategies for handling different listening environments. Some people need control of their hearing aid for the following reasons: the automatic feature does not meet their needs in 100 percent of listening situations; psychologically, these hearing aid wearers simply must have control of their hearing aids; or they are long-term hearing aid wearers habituated to a volume control and are therefore unwilling to part with it.

It's very important that you determine your needs with respect to control of the hearing aid. You don't want to fiddle with your hearing aids every ten minutes, but then again you don't want to be frustrated because your hearing aids work well in most situations but not in ten percent of your favorite situations (e.g., listening to soft music). You need to explore this topic with your hearing health professional.

7. Sound Quality

One of the most important aspects of an enjoyable hearing aid experience is that you like the sound quality of hearing aids. So when you test-run your hearing aids, make sure that you consider the following dimensions of sound quality:

- Do you like the sound of your voice?
- Is the sound clean and crisp (sound clarity)?
- Is the sound too tinny?
- Does your hearing aid plug up your ears and muffle sound?
- Does it make some pleasant soft sounds audible to you?
- Are loud sounds uncomfortable to you?
- Are your hearing aids natural sounding?
- Does music sound pleasant and rich in texture?
- Does the world sound like you're in a barrel?
- Does your hearing aid whistle, buzz, or squeal on its own?

With today's modern digital hearing aids, most of these problems should be solved. If you notice any of these problems during the trial run and in your follow-up visits, by all means talk to your hearing healthcare professional about these issues. Such professionals are now capable of adjusting your hearing aids to your satisfaction. The extent to which all of the possible sound quality issues can be resolved, of course, depends on the severity of your hearing loss. In other words, some types of hearing losses are simply more conducive to restoration of rich sound quality in many listening environments while others are not.

8. Do Not Purchase Based Only on Cosmetics

Since the 1990s, the hearing aid industry has reduced the size of hearing aids to near invisibility especially with CICs and open fit hearing aids. Some people concerned with cosmetics prefer the least noticeable hearing aids, in the same way that they might choose contact lenses instead of framed eyeglasses. The problem is that the smallest hearing aid may not be the most suitable hearing solution for you for a variety of reasons. Your specific hearing loss may require more power than is available in CICs or open fit hearing aids.

Because of hearing loss stigma or embarrassment, many consumers come into hearing healthcare offices and start off the dialog with, "I would like one of those invisible hearing aids that I saw on TV." A likely response may be something like, "We carry invisible hearing aids, but I first need to examine your ears, measure your hearing loss, assess your lifestyle and manual dexterity, and then discuss how your hearing loss is impacting the quality of your life. You may or may not be a candidate for these invisible hearing aids." If it's determined that you're not a candidate for these hearing aids, but you still insist on buying them, ethical hearing health providers will not fit you with the product because in essence they would be giving you the wrong prescription for your hearing loss.

9. Have Realistic Expectations during the Trial Period

The instructions you receive during the initial stages of adjustment are designed to help you formulate realistic expectations of what to expect from your hearing aids. You may need a specific wearing schedule for hearing aids. One experienced in-the-canal hearing aid wearer obtained CIC instruments a few years ago. He was in his early 30s and had used hearing aids since he was a teenager. When he returned for his recheck, he was asked how long he could wear the instruments in the beginning. He said that he could only use them for fifteen minutes at a time. Within two weeks, he was wearing them full-time, and they were completely comfortable. Had he not been counseled that adjusting to the deep insertion of the shell tip with CIC hearing aids may take extra time, he might have become discouraged and given up on that particular style of hearing aids.

Be patient with yourself. If you have the best hearing aids for your hearing loss and your lifestyle, hang in there. Make sure you're comfortable with the advice you've been given. Ask questions. Remember, your provider is your advocate. Satisfied hearing aid wearers are not shy when it comes to telling others about their success, but unfortunately, neither are the dissatisfied. No two people are alike, so don't assume if someone else has had a bad experience, all hearing aids are bad. You could very well be one of the overwhelming majority who has a good experience! There are many reasons why someone else may not have been successful, so don't project these conditions and improbabilities onto yourself. Also, do not expect someone else's hearing aids to work for you. Would you try on another person's eyeglasses and then decide whether you could be helped based on this experience?

Be realistic. Hearing aids will not permit you to hear the flapping of hummingbird wings over a lawnmower. Remember that it takes time to get used to hearing aids, especially if you're a new wearer.

Keep in mind that background noise is almost always part of your environment, and adjustment to it is required. In time, you'll tune out many of these everyday sounds. It's important not to become disappointed or frustrated while your brain begins to adjust to a whole new world of sound. If you're an experienced wearer trying new hearing aids, understand that they might not sound like your old ones. Before you reject them, allow neural hook-ups in the auditory system to adapt to these new sounds. You just might find that you like this new sound better than the old one.

Later on in this chapter, I'll list what I've learned you should realistically expect from your hearing aids.

10. Earwax Protection

One of the common causes of hearing aid failure is moisture and earwax filling up the receiver tubing of the hearing aid, causing the speaker to malfunction.

I strongly suggest that you purchase hearing aids with proven methods of keeping earwax out of the hearing aid. I've personally studied more than 90,000 hearing aid owners over a two-year period and determined that it's possible to reduce hearing aid repairs due to receiver failure by 50 percent by using a wax guard at the end of the hearing aids.[10]

11. Counseling and Aural Rehabilitation

I would be oversimplifying the consumer journey with hearing aids if I stated that hearing loss rehabilitation involves only being fitted with hearing aids. Some people with hearing loss will visit a hearing health professional, be tested, and then be fitted with their hearing aids, and thereby they derive optimal benefit. But many people, especially those who have delayed a solution for 10 or 15 years or who have more serious hearing losses, may need more help.

Less experienced hearing aid users should consider attending one-on-one or group sessions with their hearing health professional or doing independent study. If your hearing health professional does not offer aural rehabilitation (commonly comprising group discussion of hearing issues), by all means find a local group in your area that provides such training. A good starting point is to contact the Hearing Loss Association of America (www.shhh.org) to see if there's a self-help group in your area. The core of such training is well presented by Dr. Ross in Chapter 4. In addition, the Better Hearing Institute has provided a number of articles on the following topics (www.betterhearing.org under "Hearing Solutions"): resolution of any negative feelings you have about your hearing loss; care and maintenance of your hearing aids; communication strategies including assertiveness training; clear speech communication; and if necessary, speechreading tips for hearing in noise; your legal rights; and using computer software to retrain your auditory skills (e.g., LACE).

12. Assistive Listening Devices

For some people, especially those with severe hearing loss, hearing aids are not enough. Your hearing health professional will guide you through the array of technologies to further assist you to hear in the world. These devices may be FM hearing aids, companion microphones, bluetooth technology, telecoils for better hearing on the phone or for public places which are inductively looped, amplified telephones, specialized alarm clocks, and lamps which alert you better to your environment. If you have a telecoil in your hearing aid, by all means consider inductive looping your home so that you can hear your TV (and any other audio devices) directly into your hearing aid. (For more information on assistive listening technology, see Chapter 5 and visit www.betterhearing.org under "Hearing Solutions / Assistive Listening Devices.")

Twelve Reasons to Purchase Two Hearing Aids Instead of One

Research with more than 5,000 consumers with hearing loss in both ears demonstrated that binaurally fit subjects (with two hearing aids) were more satisfied than those monaurally fit (with one hearing aid).[12-13]

When given the choice and allowed to hear binaurally, the overwhelming majority of consumers (86 percent) chose two hearing aids over one.[1] Consequently, binaural users tend to communicate better in their place of worship, in small group gatherings, large gatherings, and even outdoors. Naturally, a person's ability to enjoy hearing aids will depend on the specific hearing loss and the type of technology used in the hearing aids.

Nevertheless, if you have a hearing loss in both ears and there is usable hearing in your poorer ear, budget permitting, I would recommend a hearing aid for both ears. Many hearing healthcare providers can demonstrate the binaural advantage on your very first visit, under headphone testing.

Based on a review of the literature and my own research with thousands of consumers with hearing loss in both ears, here are many reasons why you should consider a binaural hearing system when they're indicated.

1. Keeps both ears active, resulting in less hearing deterioration. As Dr. Carmen identifies in Chapter 1, research has shown that when only one hearing instrument is worn, the unaided ear tends to lose its ability to hear and understand. This is clinically called the *auditory deprivation effect*. People wearing two hearing instruments keep both ears active. In fact, wearing one hearing aid (when two are indicated) could result in greater deterioration of hearing in the unaided ear than if the person wore no hearing aid at all.

2. Better understanding of speech. Wearing two hearing instruments rather than one achieves selective listening more easily. Research shows that people wearing two hearing aids routinely understand speech and conversation significantly better than people wearing only one.

3. Better understanding in group and noisy situations. Wearing two hearing aids improves speech intelligibility in difficult listening situations. However, binaural digital technology tends to perform better in noise than older (analog) technologies.

4. Better ability to tell direction of sound. This is called localization. Research shows that in binaural use, there's an average of a 15 percent shift in increased satisfaction in "ability to tell the direction of sounds." This is a substantial improvement! In a social gathering, for example, localization allows you to hear from which direction someone is speaking to you. In traffic, you can tell from which direction a car or siren is coming.

5. Better sound quality. When you listen to a stereo system, you use both speakers to get the smoothest, sharpest, most natural sound quality. The same thing can be said of hearing aids. By wearing two hearing instruments, you increase your hearing range from 180 degrees reception (with just one instrument) to 360 degrees. This greater range provides a better sense of balance and sound quality.

6. Smoother tone quality. Wearing two hearing instruments generally requires less volume. This results in less distortion and more acceptable reproduction of sounds.

7. Reduced feedback and whistling. A lower volume control setting reduces the chances of feedback.

8. Wider hearing range. It's true. A person can hear sounds from a further distance with two ears, rather than just one. A voice that's barely heard at ten feet with one ear can be heard up to forty feet with two ears.

9. Better sound identification. Often, with just one hearing instrument, many noises and words sound alike. But with two hearing instruments, as with two ears, sounds are more easily distinguishable.

10. Hearing is less tiring and listening more pleasant. More binaural hearing aid wearers reported that listening and participating in conversation are more enjoyable with two instruments. This is because you do not have to strain to hear with the better ear. Thus, binaural hearing can help make listening (and therefore life) more pleasant and relaxing.

11. Feeling of balanced hearing. Two-eared hearing results in a feeling of balanced reception of sound, also known as the stereo effect, whereas monaural hearing creates an unusual feeling of sounds being heard in one ear.

12. Tinnitus Masking. About 50 percent of people with ringing in their ears reported improvement when wearing hearing aids. If you have a hearing aid in only one ear, there will still be ringing in the unaided ear.

How to Align Your Expectations with Hearing Aid Performance

Satisfaction with your hearing aids is highly dependent on the expectations you have. If you have unrealistic expectations, you'll be dissatisfied. Here are some issues you should keep in mind as you develop appropriate expectations about what your hearing aids can and cannot do for you.

- No matter how technically advanced, in most cases hearing aids cannot restore your hearing to normal except in some very mild hearing losses.
- Not all hearing aids perform the same with every type of hearing loss.
- No hearing aid will filter out all background noise. Some hearing instruments can reduce amplification of some types of background noise or make you more comfortable in the presence of noise.

- Where appropriate, directional microphones can often improve your ability to hear in noise.
- Directional hearing instruments coupled with digital signal processing will optimize your hearing instruments for improving your quality of life in noisy environments.
- Since you're purchasing custom hearing instruments, you should expect the fit to be comfortable; ideally you should not even know they're in your ears. There should not be any soreness, bleeding, or rashes associated with wearing hearing aids. If there is, go back to your hearing health provider to make adjustments to the shell of the aid or earmold.
- Hearing instruments should allow you to:
  (1) hear soft sounds (e.g., child's voice, soft speech) that you couldn't hear without amplification—this is part of the enjoyment of hearing aids;
  (2) understand speech in quiet situations—many people will derive some additional speech intelligibility in noise with advanced technology;
  (3) prevent loud sounds from becoming uncomfortably loud for you, but very loud sounds that are uncomfortable to normal hearing people may still be uncomfortable to you.
- Hearing aids may squeal or whistle when you're inserting them into your ear (if you don't have a volume control to shut it off); but if the aid squeals after the initial insertion, then most likely you have an inadequate fit and should tell your hearing health provider.
- Do not expect your friend's hearing aid brand or style to work for you.
- Do not expect your family doctor to know very much about hearing loss, brands of hearing aids, and your need for them.
- Expect your hearing aids to provide benefit to you during the trial period. By benefit, I mean that your ability to understand speech has demonstrably improved in the listening situations important to you (with realistic expectations though). This is what you paid for, so you should expect benefit. If you don't experience an improvement, then work with your hearing health professional to adjust the instrument to meet your specific needs. Never purchase a hearing aid that does not give you sufficient benefit.
- Expect to be satisfied with your hearing instruments and expect the quality of your life to improve.

- Expect a 30-day trial period with a money-back guarantee if your hearing aids do not give you benefit. (There might be a small nonrefundable portion for some services rendered.)
- Give your hearing aids a chance, being sure to follow the instructions of the hearing health provider. Most people need a period of adjustment (called acclimatization) before they're deriving maximum benefit (even up to four months).

Common Myths about Hearing Loss and Hearing Aids

There are many common myths still prevalent about hearing loss and hearing aids. I would like to dispel these myths now that you're living in the 21st Century.

"My hearing loss cannot be helped."

In the past, many people with hearing loss in one ear, with a high frequency hearing loss, or with nerve damage have all been told they cannot be helped, often by their family practice physician. This might have been true many years ago, but with modern advances in technology, nearly 95 percent of people with a sensorineural hearing loss <u>can</u> benefit from hearing aids.

"Hearing loss affects only <u>old people</u> and is <u>a sign of aging</u>."

Only 35 percent of people with hearing loss are older than age 64. There are close to six million people in the U.S. between the ages of 18 and 44 with hearing loss, and more than one million are of school age. Hearing loss affects all age groups.

"If I had a hearing loss, my family doctor would have told me. "

Not true! Only 13 percent of physicians routinely screen for hearing loss during a physical. Since most hard of hearing people hear well in a quiet environment like your doctor's office, it can be virtually impossible for your physician to recognize the extent of your problem. Without special training in and understanding of the nature of hearing loss, it may be difficult for your doctor to even believe that you have a hearing problem.

"The consequences of hiding hearing loss are better than wearing hearing aids."

What price are you paying for vanity? I go back to the old adage that an untreated hearing loss is far more noticeable than hearing aids. If you miss a punch line to a joke or respond inappropriately in conversation, people may have concerns about your mental acuity, your attention span, or your ability to communicate effectively. The personal consequences of vanity can be life altering. At a simplistic level, untreated hearing loss means giving up some of the pleasant sounds you used to enjoy. At a deeper level, vanity could severely reduce the quality of your life.

"Only people with serious hearing loss need hearing aids."

The need for hearing amplification is dependent on your lifestyle, your need for refined hearing, and the degree of your hearing loss. If you're a lawyer, teacher, or a group psychotherapist, where very acute hearing is necessary to discern the nuances of human communication, then even a mild hearing loss can be intolerable. If you live in a rural area by yourself and seldom socialize, then perhaps you're someone who is tolerant of your hearing loss.

"I'll just have some minor surgery like my friend did, and then my hearing will be okay."

Many people know someone whose hearing improved after medical or surgical treatment, and it's true that some types of hearing loss can be successfully treated. With adults, unfortunately, this only applies to five to ten percent of cases.

"My hearing loss is normal for my age."

Isn't this a strange way to look at things? But, do you realize that well-meaning physicians tell this to their patients every day? It happens to be "normal" for overweight people to have high blood pressure or diabetes. That doesn't mean they should not receive treatment for the problem.

"I have one ear that's down a little, but the other one's okay."

Everything is relative. Nearly all patients who believe that they have one "good" ear actually have two "bad" ears. When one ear is slightly better than the other, we learn to favor that ear for the telephone, group conversations, and so forth. It can give the illusion that "the better ear" is normal when it isn't. Most types of hearing loss affect both ears fairly equally, and about 90 percent of patients are in need of hearing aids for both ears.

Hearing aids will make me <u>look older</u> or <u>handicapped</u>."

Looking older is clearly more affected by almost all other factors besides hearing aids. It's not the hearing aids that make one look older, it's the way you conduct yourself in the absence of hearing aids.

If hearing aids help you function like a normal hearing person, for all intents and purposes, the stigma is removed. Hearing aid manufacturers are well aware that cosmetics are an issue to many people, and that's why today we have hearing aids that fit totally in the ear canal (essentially not noticeable unless someone is staring directly into your ear). These CIC and open fit styles of hearing aids have enough power and special features to satisfy at least half of individuals with hearing loss. But more importantly, worth repeating is that untreated hearing loss is more obvious than a hearing aid. Smiling and nodding your head when you don't understand what's being said make your condition more apparent than the largest hearing aid.

"Hearing aids will make everything sound too loud."

Hearing aids are amplifiers. At one time, the way hearing aids were designed, it was necessary to turn up the power in order to hear soft speech (or other soft sounds). With today's hearing aids, the circuit works automatically, only providing the amplification needed based on the input level. In fact, many hearing aids today don't have a volume control.

Conclusions

Hopefully, you now recognize the value of hearing aids and the significant impact they can have on your life, as well as the life of your family, loved ones and associates. I also hope you realize that hearing aids may not necessarily be an instant cure for your hearing difficulties, but with patience, you'll find they can be your bridge to healing. Enjoy the experience!

References

1. Kochkin,S. (2005) MarkeTrak VII: Hearing loss population tops 31 million people. *The Hearing Review* 12(7):16-29.
2. Kochkin S. (2000) MarkeTrak V: Why my hearing aids are in the drawer: the consumer's perspective. *The Hearing Journal* 53(2):34-42.
3. Kochkin S. (2007) MarkeTrak VII: Obstacles to adult non-user adoption of hearing aids. *The Hearing Journal* 60(4):27-43.
4. Kochkin S. (2005) Customer satisfaction with hearing aids in the Digital Age. *The Hearing Journal* 58(9):30-37.
5. Kochkin S. (1996) Customer satisfaction and subjective benefit with high-performance hearing instruments. *The Hearing Review* 3(12):16-26.

6. Kochkin S. (2006) Thin-tube BTE survey. Washington, DC: Better Hearing Institute.

7. Kochkin S and Rogin C. (2000) Quantifying the obvious: the impact of hearing aids on quality of life, *The Hearing Review* 7(1):8-34.

8. Singer J, Healey J and Preece J. (1997) Hearing instruments: a psychological and behavioral perspective. *High Performance Hearing Solutions* 1:23-27.

9. Kochkin S. (2000) Customer satisfaction with single and multiple microphone digital hearing aids, *The Hearing Review* 7(11):24-29.

10. Kochkin S. (2002) Finally a solution to the cerumen problem. *The Hearing Review* 9(4):46-49.

12. Kochkin S and Kuk F. (1997) The binaural advantage: evidence from subjective benefit and customer satisfaction data. *The Hearing Review* 4(4):29,30-32,34.

13. Kochkin S. (2000) Binaural hearing aids: the fitting of choice for bilateral loss subjects. (An unpublished technical paper.) Itasca, IL: Knowles Electronics.

14. Allen R. (2002) Reasonable expectations for the consumer. www.healthy hearing.com. August.

15. Stypulkowski P. (1997) Realistic expectations: a key to success. *High Performance Hearing Solutions* 1:56-57.

CHAPTER THREE
Hearing Aid Technology
And Rehabilitation

Robert W. Sweetow, Ph.D.

Dr. Sweetow is Director of Audiology and Professor in the Department of Otolaryngology at the University of California, San Francisco. He received his Ph.D. from Northwestern University in 1977. He holds a Master of Arts degree from the University of Southern California and a Bachelor of Science degree from the University of Iowa. Dr. Sweetow has lectured worldwide, and has authored 25 textbook chapters and over 100 scientific articles on counseling, tinnitus, aural rehabilitation and amplification for the hearing impaired. He recently developed an interactive training program for Listening and Communication Enhancement (LACE) that is designed for home use.

There are many myths and misconceptions regarding hearing aids. The objective of this chapter is to prepare you with accurate up-to-date information to help in your decision to upgrade or try new hearing aids. Keeping up to date is very important, and sometimes difficult to do because technology is changing so rapidly. But in today's world, consumers need to be educated so that they can work together with their professional to make the best decisions possible. This chapter addresses questions you may ask yourself before and even during your test drive of hearing aids.

"Am I a candidate for hearing aids?"

Forty years ago, many hearing healthcare professionals believed that only people with hearing loss due to outer or middle ear problems (conductive hearing loss) could be helped by hearing aids. Patients were often told that hearing aids could make sounds <u>louder</u> (like turning up the volume on a radio), but would not necessarily make sounds <u>clearer</u>. This thinking was reinforced by reports of unfavorable results from those hard of hearing patients who did try hearing aids and who still couldn't understand speech clearly— particularly in noisy places. Of course, it's now recognized that early attempts to fit hearing aids on people with nerve damage (sensorineural hearing loss) were seriously hindered by the limited sound quality produced by these early devices; by the limited choice of electronic variations; and by inadequate fitting strategies used in trying to determine the best manner to amplify speech without making it too loud or too noisy.

In the early days of fitting hearing aids, professionals often tried to determine who was a candidate on the basis of the degree of hearing loss shown on the hearing test. Simply considering the degree of hearing loss, however isn't adequate to describe the impact hearing loss has on your life. Indeed, it oversimplifies the complexities of hearing impairment. By using a more "holistic" approach to identifying and correcting communication difficulties, not just hearing loss, we realize that candidacy is based more on your communicative <u>needs</u> rather than purely on test results obtained in a sound booth. Your own personal *subjective needs* are what matters. A good litmus test is to ask yourself whether you feel stressed or fatigued after a day of straining to hear. Hearing aids may simply relieve this strain, rather than making sounds louder or allowing you to understand all speech in all listening environments. Reducing strain alone can be very important, not only to you, but to those trying to talk to you. Therefore, *properly fitted hearing aids can provide benefit even if you have a relatively mild hearing loss.*

It was also incorrectly believed that you couldn't use hearing aids if you had normal hearing for low-pitched sounds (up to 1500 or 2000 Hz); if you had a hearing loss in only one ear; if your speech understanding abilities were reduced; or if you had difficulty tolerating loud sounds (for example, a crying baby). Advances in technology now allow for good fittings for most patients experiencing these problems.

Occupational and social demands vary greatly among individuals. A judge who has a mild hearing loss may desperately need amplification, while a retired person living alone with the exact same degree of hearing loss may not. You must unselfishly examine whether you're becoming a burden to others, even if you do not personally recognize difficulty hearing. *Remember that wearing hearing aids may be a symbol of courtesy to others.*

Unfortunately, despite need, many people resist trying hearing aids. There are three main reasons for this resistance.

First is *hearsay*. A lot of us have friends or relatives who have purchased hearing aids that currently reside in their dresser drawers. These unsuccessful wearers of amplification are more than happy to spread the gospel on the limitations (some accurate, some not) of hearing aids. Often, unsuccessful experiences occurred in extremely difficult listening environments in which even people with normal hearing had trouble understanding speech.

Second, despite the fact that people of all ages have hearing impairment and use amplification, there has been an undeniable *social stigma* attached to wearing hearing aids. The problem of vanity has been eased, in large part, by the continuing trend toward hearing devices that can barely be seen. However, not all listeners with hearing loss are candidates for these devices.

The third reason is the perception that *the relatively high cost of hearing aids is not reflected in the value and benefits they provide.* This is a valid concern, so when making a decision as to whether this is the right time for you to try hearing aids, you must weigh whether the financial investment can be offset by the improvement in your quality of life by reducing your hearing difficulty. Be sure to consider improvements from a social, emotional, and occupational perspective, and remember to consider activities you'd like to undertake but have given up because of communication difficulties.

It's a double-edged sword when it comes to dispensing hearing aids to a person who's not motivated to wear amplification. On one hand, a poorly motivated person is not the best candidate for amplification regardless of the degree of hearing loss. So, from this perspective, the answer to the question of whether a steadfastly reluctant person should be forced into trying a hearing aid is probably *no*. If you're absolutely opposed to trying hearing aids at this time, and if you're convinced you'll fail, it may be advisable to wait until another time when you may be more optimistic about the process.

On the other hand, keep in mind that it's <u>very</u> <u>possible</u> you'll be pleasantly surprised. Remember that, as will be discussed later in this chapter, there have been more changes in hearing aids during the last few years than in the previous forty.

"How do hearing aids work?"

As I stated at the beginning of this chapter, hearing aids have dramatically changed. Until the mid 1990's, hearing aids contained four or five basic components. Sound would enter the hearing aid through a tiny <u>microphone</u>. This sound was then converted to an electrical current which was fed into an <u>amplifier</u> and filtered by electrical components that established how much relative amplification would be provided for the different frequencies. For example, most hearing aids try to amplify the high pitches more than the low pitches. The overall amount of amplification, for most, but not all, hearing aids was then governed by a <u>volume control</u>. The newly formed amplified electrical signal was then sent to a <u>receiver</u>, also called a loudspeaker. The receiver converted the electrical signal back into sound waves that exit the hearing aid and enter the ear canal through the <u>earmold</u> for Behind-The-Ear (BTE) hearing aids, or through a tube inside the plastic shell for In-The-Ear (ITE) styles. Also, all hearing aids are run by a tiny <u>battery</u>, which generally lasts for between one to three weeks.

"Are digital hearing aids better than analog?"

The amplification of sound just described was done using analog hearing aids. In the mid 1990s the first generation of digital hearing aids was introduced. A digital hearing aid has a computer chip performing the signal processing and amplification steps instead of the traditional "analog" circuitry described above. It's actually a miniature computer in itself. This is a major breakthrough in technology because it greatly increases the amount of sound processing possible in the given amount of space. Digital hearing aids tend to have minimal distortion, advanced feedback control, improved noise suppression, and better control over the directional or multiple microphones. They have the ability to analyze the sound environment and adapt amplification accordingly, typically making speech clearer. They also can recognize the difference between the human voice versus incoming noise to further improve speech perception. This is all done automatically without the need for volume or remote controls. In addition, they allow for greater flexibility for the professional to program. We will talk about each of these features later.

"What hearing aid styles are appropriate for me?"

In the early 1950s, you would have been limited to a choice of two styles of hearing instruments: body borne or in-eyeglass frames. These devices are almost never seen today. Now, however, you have many options regarding hearing aid styles (see Figure 3-1). BTE hearing aids (sometimes called Over-the-Ear or OTE) sit over the outer ear and are connected to an earpiece or earmold located in the concha (bowl) of the ear and ear canal. BTE aids come in variety of sizes.

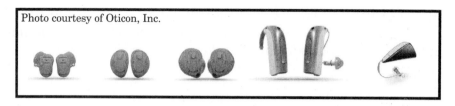

Photo courtesy of Oticon, Inc.

Figure 3-1: Hearing devices (left to right): pair of CICs, pair of ITCs, pair of ITEs, BTE (without earmold), BTE open fit with thin tubing and ear tip, and on far right is a Receiver-In-The-Ear (RITE) hearing device

There are a number of options regarding the earpiece that directs the sound into your ear. Some completely fill the ear canal, while others allow for air (and sound) to get directly into the ear canal without being amplified. These latter devices are called *open fit* hearing aids. They came onto the market in 2004 and have become extremely popular since they're comfortable, barely visible (unless you have no hair), and can often be fit immediately because they often don't require a custom-made earmold.

The other main style of hearing aids is the custom in-the-ear (ITE). These devices include the full shell, which completely fills the bowl and ear canal); the thinner low profile; the partially occluding half concha; the in-the-canal (ITC); and the tiniest of ITE hearing aids, the completely-in-canal (CIC).

While cosmetic considerations may be important, the decision as to which style hearing aid is most appropriate for you should be based on both <u>physical</u> as well as <u>audiological</u> factors.

"What are the physical factors that can influence fitting of my hearing aids?"

Anatomical characteristics may dictate the style; for example, BTE hearing aids may not be able to be used if you have deformed outer ears; the depth of your concha may determine the suitability of ITE model instruments; and in order to be able to wear the ITC or CIC type instruments, your ear canal must not be so curvy that it prevents easy insertion and removal.

Manual dexterity is important in handling hearing aids. Not only is removal and insertion of hearing aids somewhat difficult for certain people, but the ability to manipulate controls and the battery must be considered and assessed before you decide that a certain style is right for you. Always ask your hearing professional to show you the different styles, and if possible, to let you try these devices prior to purchasing. Keep in mind, however, that this sometimes takes a little practice, so don't get discouraged if you can't insert or remove the hearing aid from your ear, or the battery from the hearing aid the first time you try.

Some people need hearing aids that are large enough to accommodate a vent (hole) drilled into it, so that air can enter your ear canal. Without this *ventilation*, you may perceive a "plugged up" feeling or you may sound to yourself like you're "in a barrel" when you speak. This phenomenon is called the "occlusion effect." You may demonstrate this to yourself by sticking your finger in your ear and counting out loud. People who have similar hearing in each ear and who have nerve damage will find that their own voice shifts toward the blocked ear. This happens because normally when we vocalize, our ear canal vibrates and this vibration leaks out of the ear and into the air without being noticed. But when you block your ear, as some hearing aids might do, the vibration gets trapped in your ear canal and you sound like you're in a barrel. Some people find CIC hearing aids are particularly prone to the "occlusion effect." Also, for some people, CIC hearing aids can be uncomfortable because they may extend deeply into the ear canal and may be physically uncomfortable to you because the skin is much thinner than it is at the outer part of the canal.

Some styles of hearing aid, particularly the open fit OTE devices that are attached to non-occluding ear pieces (those that don't block your ear canals) may be more comfortable to wear and don't create this occlusion effect. In addition, if your ears produce excessive cerumen (earwax), or are very hairy, you may be better off with BTE rather than ITE devices.

Medical Contraindications such as draining ears or other medical problems may prevent the use of any hearing aid apparatus blocking your ear canals. In this instance, you'll need open, non-occluding earmolds or possibly bone conduction-type systems. This latter type of hearing aid is beyond the scope of this discussion, but can be reviewed by your hearing healthcare provider if applicable to you.

"What audiological factors will influence my fitting?"

The *audiometric pattern* on your audiogram may show certain frequencies (pitches) that have normal hearing. For example, if you have a high frequency hearing loss but have normal hearing in the low frequencies, you may be best served by systems that are non-occluding (see below) and thus allow low-pitched sounds to pass into your ear without being amplified. Conversely, if you have a hearing loss in the low frequencies, it is necessary to keep low frequency amplification in your ear, so a hearing aid that fills the ear canal may be necessary.

The *degree of loss* may predict the need for a specific kind of hearing aid. For example, severe and profound hearing losses are best served by BTE-style hearing aids with full earmolds. A mild loss however, can use almost any style of hearing aid.

Special features may be important for you, such as directional or multiple microphones (which primarily amplify signals coming from in front of you and will be discussed later) and/or the addition of a telecoil (a magnetic induction loop). Telecoils allow sound to bypass the hearing aid microphone and amplify signals received electro-magnetically (from telephones). In addition to allowing you to listen on the telephone without feedback (whistling), telecoils can interface with a variety of assistive listening devices. At the time of this writing, CIC hearing aids are simply too small to contain these special features.

On the other hand, one advantage of CIC hearing aids is that the microphone lies either within, or at the entrance of the ear canal and thus is able to benefit fully from the *natural amplification* of the outer ear bowl. The receiver of the hearing aid is located closer to the eardrum, where the amount of air trapped in the ear canal that needs to vibrate is less than for most other fittings. Therefore, *less hearing aid amplification is needed* to produce the same sound pressure at the eardrum. This often results in lower distortion levels.

Because of this advantage, and given the possible discomfort or occlusion from CICs, many of the open fit BTEs now separate the microphone (which is housed in the BTE part of the hearing aid), from the receiver (loudspeaker) which is contained in the ear canal. These devices are called Receiver in the Ear, or RITE hearing aids.

Acoustic feedback refers to the whistling or ringing sound often produced when you cup your hand or hold a telephone over your ear while wearing a hearing aid. It also occurs when the hearing aid or earmold is not properly or snugly inserted in your ear. It happens because the sound amplified by the hearing aid leaks out of your ear canal and goes back through the microphone of the hearing aid and is re-amplified. Feedback from hearing aids can be annoying not only to you, but to others. It's not acceptable, except momentarily when covering your ear or inserting the device into your ear. The more amplification that is required (because of your degree of hearing loss), the more likely it is that feedback could occur. Generally speaking, the closer the microphone where the sound enters) is to the exit point of the amplified sound from the hearing aid or earmold, the greater the likelihood of feedback. BTE hearing aids often have an advantage over smaller ITE or ITC styles in this regard since there's more physical distance between the microphone and the receiver. However, if you use an open fit BTE that doesn't block your ear, there is a big opening through which amplified sound can leak back into the microphone. Advanced digital hearing aids contain "active feedback management" systems. An active system detects feedback and counteracts it before it occurs by creating "counter signals" to cancel or at least minimize the feedback.

In any case, it's important that the earmolds or hearing aid shells fit perfectly in your ears. This is why it's essential that your hearing healthcare professional takes good impressions of your ears before you obtain hearing aids. If you haven't yet had an earmold impression taken, don't worry. It doesn't hurt. Your provider will first place a cotton or foam block in your ear canal and then inject liquid material in your ear that will harden in about five minutes. It's a similar process to getting impressions made by the dentist, except thankfully, you don't need a Novocain shot!

It's not unusual to find that the most important factors determining success or failure of a fitting are those unrelated to audiometric findings. In particular, you must take into consideration all of the following: your age and general physical and mental health; your motivation (as opposed to that of your family's); finances; cosmetic considerations; and your communication needs. It's heartening to note that the primary reasons for rejection of hearing aids, after people try them, are less related to finances and cosmetics, and have more to do with difficulty hearing in background noise, and discomfort from loud sounds. These problems are well on the way to being lessened by modern-day hearing aids and fitting techniques.

"How do I adjust the volume so that I can hear soft sounds and so that loud sounds don't overwhelm me?"

A lot of people don't realize that when you have a hearing loss due to nerve damage (sensorineural), your hearing problem is primarily limited to difficulty hearing soft sounds. Your ability to hear loud sounds may be okay. In fact, many people with sensorineural hearing loss find louder sounds to be uncomfortable. So, there are three basic rules that must be followed if a hearing aid fitting is to be successful: soft sounds must be made audible (so that you can hear them); normal conversational sounds must be comfortable; loud sounds must not be uncomfortable.

The way to achieve this goal is with a technique called *compression*. Here is how it works: In the past, hearing aids would provide the same amount of amplification to soft incoming sounds as they would for loud incoming sounds. The technical term for this is *linear* amplification. This would allow people to hear the soft sounds but the loud sounds would then be uncomfortable or even painful. So, many wearers reported that in order to hear soft sounds, they had to turn their hearing aids up too high. This did indeed allow them to hear soft sounds but it also produced the undesirable effect of making loud sounds uncomfortable. Here's why: Imagine that a certain level of sound enters the hearing aid, let's say 65 dB (which happens to be about the level of normal conversational speech). To make this speech comfortable, the volume of the hearing aid might be set so that it produces 25 dB of amplification. Therefore, 90 dB comes into the ear canal (65 plus 25). Now, lets imagine that the sound coming into the hearing aid suddenly becomes much louder, as might occur in a restaurant when people at your table start to laugh at a joke. If you're wearing a linear aid, the sound coming into it is now increased to 80 dB, and this type of hearing aid will still add 25 dB of amplification, so the sound in your ear canal increases to 105 dB. For most people, this will be entirely too loud and uncomfortable, and your reaction will be to try and turn it down using the volume control. This is why you might have seen people with linear hearing aids adjusting the volume control quite often when sound intensity in the surrounding environment changed.

In 1992, a new type of hearing aid was introduced using more advanced technology called *non-linear*, or *dynamic range compression*. With this, there's more amplification given to soft sounds than there is for louder sounds. In other words, when sounds are above a certain level set in the hearing aid, it's as if an invisible finger reaches up and automatically moves the volume down for you, and vice versa, when the sound environment becomes lower than a certain level it moves the volume up for you.

This type of non-linear hearing aid basically squeezes a wide range of loudness into a narrower range, which has generated the other descriptive name of *compression hearing aids*. Going back to the earlier example, now with the non-linear type, when sounds entering the hearing aid suddenly increase to 80 dB, the amplification may be automatically lowered from 25 dB to 10 dB. Therefore, the sound reaching your eardrum is a more comfortable 90 dB as opposed to the uncomfortable 105.

There were two big problems with this early form of compression. The first was that when loud sounds would enter the hearing aid microphone, it would trigger a change in amplification such that *all* sounds were reduced to maintain comfort. This was called *single channel compression*. The problem with this is that an individual's loudness growth pattern may be different from one pitch to another. That is, you might find that high-pitched sounds (like dishes clanging) seem painfully loud to you but low-pitched sounds (a refrigerator humming) do not. Therefore, the amount of compression needed to be different for various frequencies. This is where the next step up in circuitry sophistication comes in, *non-linear multiple channel compression*. Hearing aids with multiple channels can divide the incoming signal into as few as three, or as many over twenty channels.

With multiple channel compression, characteristics of the hearing aid will be tailored to your personal needs based upon how loud you interpret certain sounds to be for various frequencies. Perhaps there will be a lot of compression for the high frequencies but very little for the low frequencies. Compression helps to make sounds appear comfortably loud for you.

The second thing multichannel compression accomplishes may be even more important. If your hearing aid system has only one channel, a loud noise made up of mostly low frequencies (as might be found in cocktail parties) would instruct the hearing aid that it needs to lower its amplification for all frequencies. This would help to keep the sound from being too loud, but it would make some of the high frequency sounds (like consonants) too soft to hear. On the other hand, a multichannel hearing aid, in that same loud low frequency noise situation, would decrease the amplification for low frequencies, making sound comfortable without changing the amplification for the high frequencies (thus preserving audibility of important high frequency consonant sounds). This can actually produce additional high frequency amplification while simultaneously reducing low frequency amplification, all depending on the sound environment.

Non-linear, multiple channel hearing aids act not only as a means of loudness control, but also as a means of differentiating the amount of amplification given to different parts of the speech signal. If fitted correctly, they can dampen the strong elements of speech, such as vowels, and enhance the delicate speech elements such as the /s/, /sh/ and /f/ sounds. This can improve speech clarity, especially in difficult listening environments. Hearing aids containing multichannel compression can regulate themselves so automatically that they frequently don't contain a volume control. You may find this to your liking if you're the type who doesn't like to frequently adjust your hearing aids, or, you may feel that not having a volume control takes away too much control from you. This is something you should discuss carefully with your hearing healthcare provider.

"Will my hearing aids help me when I'm in background noise?"

We live in a noisy world. Many people with hearing loss correctly believe that they can hear pretty well in quiet, but as soon as there is background noise, like in a restaurant or a room with lots of people talking, their understanding is poor. The truth is, people with hearing loss typically have more trouble <u>understanding</u> speech in noise even if they can <u>hear</u> the speech than do people with normal hearing. Hearing aids in the past were not very good at separating speech from noise. The strategy was that if the hearing aid reduced the amplification for the low frequencies, where there was a lot of noise energy, you would be able to hear speech better. The problem was that while this approach might indeed reduce the loudness of the noise, it also tended to make speech softer. This occurred since speech has a lot of the same, primarily low frequency (pitch) sound energy as noise. As digital processing became more sophisticated, newer and better methods of controlling noise have emerged. One of these approaches, called *noise reduction*, works on a different principle. Even though speech and noise can have similar energy in terms of pitch, the temporal (timing) and the amplitude (loudness) characteristics of the signals are quite different. The computerized processing contained in certain hearing aids can measure and calculate these characteristics and thus determine what is speech and what is noise. Then, similar to the way multiple channel compression works, the digital processor can limit the amount of amplification for those channels (bands) that are judged to contain more noise than speech, or conversely, provide full amplification in the bands that contain more speech than noise. Noise reduction doesn't necessarily make speech clearer when it is immersed in a lot of background noise, but it can make the background seem much more comfortable.

Another approach to controlling noise might, in fact, make speech in noise clearer. Typically, you face the person who is speaking to you. Noise, however, may originate in front, behind, and/or to your sides. Many hearing aids now contain *directional* or *multiple microphones* that "communicate" with each other so that sounds originating from the front of the hearing aid receive maximum amplification, and sounds originating from the sides or behind receive less amplification. This effectively suppresses some (though not all) of the annoying background noise that may create so much difficulty for you. When you wear hearing aids with multiple microphones, you can try to position yourself in a room so that noise is less bothersome. For example, in a restaurant, you should take a seat with your back toward the center of the room where most of the noise is located, or similarly, away from the kitchen.

Of course, if you're a taxi driver, or if you need to hear children in the back seat when you're driving, you may be better off with hearing aids that amplify sounds equally from all directions. Another example of when you might want amplification to occur from all around you would be when listening to music. Some hearing aids allow you to select whether you want most of the amplification to occur for signals in front of you or whether you want equal amplification for signals all around you. Also, some of the hearing aids will allow you to touch a button on the hearing aid or in a remote control that will turn on the directional function, while others will automatically turn on this function automatically whenever it detects noise. Another exciting new feature using multiple microphones is that the directional function can be adaptive. This means that not only will the hearing aid automatically switch into the directional mode, but it will determine exactly where the noise is coming from and specifically target those directions for a reduction in amplification. This adaptive directionality can be especially useful considering that the location of unwanted noise is not always directly behind you and is certainly not always coming from the same direction.

It's also important to know that multiple microphones require a minimal space requirement of at least 3 mm between the microphones. Because of their small size, CIC hearing aids are unable to accommodate this useful feature, though some natural directivity is achieved by the placement of CICs within the ear canal.

Despite these improvements, we must face the reality that some environments are simply too noisy for hard of hearing or normal hearing people to comfortably converse. In those situations, no matter how good the hearing aids are, expect to still have problems.

"I like to listen to music. Can hearing aids help?"

Hearing aids are certainly able to make musical sounds audible (capable of being heard) that you might not hear without amplification. However, if some of the same strategies that are applied to listening to speech were applied to listening to music, there might be some problems. For example, while noise reduction can be helpful for reducing unpleasant noise, your hearing aids could be "tricked" into believing that certain parts of music are noise, and would then reduce the amplification for those parts of the music. Of course, one might argue that some of the music that is heard these days really is nothing more than noise, but that is another story! So programs designed for music should not employ noise reduction. In addition, as mentioned earlier, part of the enjoyment of music is having the sounds enter each ear from a variety of directions. So here again, while multiple and directional microphones are really helpful when listening to speech, you're better off listening to music with hearing aids that amplify equally from all directions. Fortunately, most of the new hearing aids that contain the directional feature, will allow you to turn off this feature manually or will automatically do so for you. Another difference in the strategies used in hearing music as opposed to speech is that music programs don't use so much compression. The reason for this is so that the full range of musical sounds (from soft to loud) is preserved.

A limitation in hearing aids, relative to home stereo systems, is that the *bandwidth* (number of frequencies amplified by the hearing aid) is more restricted. While the bandwidth of hearing aids keeps getting wider, there are presently some limits because of the very small loudspeaker that is contained in hearing aids and the fact that hearing aids are powered by a battery that provides only a small amount of current (compared to plugging your home stereo into a wall outlet).

"How do hearing aids know which features and which programs to use?"

Once you and your hearing care provider have selected the appropriate hearing aids and features based on your communication needs, the devices may be programmed to contain multiple programs (typically two to four), that are specifically designed for different situations, such as listening in quiet, listening in noise, adjusting for comfort in constant noise (like in your car), listening to music, or listening to the telephone. You can select which program is right for different situations by pressing a button on the hearing aid or a remote control. Alternatively, you may choose to have the hearing aid work in an *automatic mode* in which it makes selection of the optimal program based on characteristics of sounds entering the hearing aid. Multiple programs can also be very useful if you have a fluctuating hearing loss such as in Ménière's disease.

"Will I be able to hear on my cell phone?"

It's very important that you're able to use the telephone with your hearing aids. Too frequently, hearing aid users believe they must remove their hearing aids when they talk on the phone because otherwise they get feedback. Not only is this annoying and embarrassing, but it makes hearing the voice at the other end of the call especially hard. To combat this problem, BTE and ITE (but not CIC) hearing aids can contain a *telecoil*, a small metal inductance coil hidden within the aid that picks up and amplifies electro-magnetic leakage produced from telephones. When the telecoil is activated, you have the option to turn off the microphone to eliminate feedback or undesirable environmental sounds. Telecoils also are used to interface with various assistive listening devices. To activate the telecoil program, you can either press a button on the aid, use a remote control, or get a hearing aid that automatically switches itself into the telecoil mode as soon as it detects electromagnetic leakage from the phone. Then, when you remove the phone from your ear, the hearing aid automatically switches back into the normal listening program.

Certain cellular phones create a buzzing static or interference if used with a hearing aid telecoil and are therefore incompatible with telecoil usage. However, recent FCC regulations have forced wireless phone manufacturers to produce more cell phone models that will work with hearing aids. It's a very good idea to find out if your hearing aid will work with a cell phone before you buy a new phone and before you purchase hearing aids. The best way to do this is to try it out first.

At least three wireless phone manufacturers including Nokia, Motorola and Ericsson have developed neckloops that can be used with a T-coil. The neckloops permit hands-free use of the cell phone, and binaural (two ear) listening if the user has two hearing aids with T-coils. The phone itself can be carried in a pocket or clipped onto clothing. Some newer hearing aids contain automatic switching into the telecoil mode, so that when you pick up the telephone and hold it to your ear, the telecoil is activated without requiring the user to switch programs. For hearing aids that don't contain telecoils, such as CICs (which are too small to house the inductance coil), the use of multiple programs can be effective by dedicating one program to a frequency response that de-emphasizes amplification in the high frequencies that might produce feedback. This works because most telephones don't transduce sounds in the very high frequencies anyway.

Be sure to tell your hearing care professional what kind of a telephone system you use. For example, if you use a Bluetooth telephone, some hearing aids can offer you a feature that will wirelessly interface your hearing aids to the Bluetooth phone. This is a very nice, wireless, hands-free feature that could actually allow you to hear the telephone in both ears. And speaking of binaural (two-eared) listening, you could even listen through your hearing aids to music downloaded onto your phone or iPod or MP3 player. (For more information on Bluetooth, cell phones and land line phones, see Chapter 5.)

"If my hearing changes are my hearing aids obsolete?"

Don't worry. Most digital hearing aids have a great amount of programming flexibility that allows your practitioner to adjust your hearing aids to a wide range, accommodating most audiometric configurations and allowing for adjustment for your individual loudness comfort levels. Of course, there are some limitations. Hearing aids appropriate for a mild or moderate degree of hearing loss won't be powerful enough for someone with a profound loss. Similarly, the style of the hearing aid may limit the fitting range. For instance, you can't use the open fit, mini BTE aids discussed earlier if you suddenly develop a substantial loss in the low frequencies.

"How will I know if I'm properly using the hearing aids and if they're properly programmed?"

A new feature that is available in some hearing aids is referred to as *datalogging*. This feature can provide your professional with information about the number of hours you wear the hearing aids, the relative amount of time you spend in each program, how often you change the controls, and even the percentage of time you spend in different acoustic environments. Some hearing aids are even considered "trainable" because they'll automatically adjust their programming based on the information obtained from the datalog. This datalogging information can be quite informative to both you and to the professional who programs your hearing aids to meet your needs.

"Is there ever going to be a disposable hearing aid?"

There have been some attempts in the past to manufacture disposable and entry-level hearing aids. A potential advantage of these devices is that your initial investment may be less and the devices may not be as susceptible to technological obsolescence because they're designed for temporary use. Thus, if after a limited period of time, you decide that the hearing aids aren't meeting your needs, they can be discarded and no further money is invested, kind of like disposable contact lenses. To date, however, none have achieved widespread acceptance due to physical comfort and ethical concerns regarding the methods with which they're dispensed to the public. Recently however, one manufacturer introduced a new device that fits halfway down the ear canal and is completely invisible. The device is designed to be worn 24 hours a day, and it lasts for between two to four months. When the instrument battery expires the entire aid is discarded and replaced with a new one by a trained hearing professional who has access to a microscope for safe insertion into the ear canal. The hearing aid is sold on an annual subscription basis. There are some restrictions on who can use this device. You must have healthy ear canals that are of the correct diameter, shape, and depth, and free of bony obstructions, skin conditions, or frequent and excessive earwax accumulation.

"What limitations might I expect with hearing aids?"

Hearing aids are meant to minimize listening fatigue and improve ease of communication. They're not meant to allow you to "hear a pin drop," and there are going to be circumstances in which hearing aids don't give you all the benefits you'd like. The most frequent complaints voiced by hearing aid wearers are that noise is overly amplified, certain sounds become too loud to bear, and some speech remains unclear.

No hearing aids effectively eliminate all background noise. If all the sound energy that makes up noise were eliminated, important segments of speech also would be missing. And, remember that normal listeners experience background noise daily. If all background noise were eliminated, the acoustic world would be quite boring and unnatural. Even so, don't hesitate to discuss your perception of background noise with your provider so that your hearing aids can be fine-tuned to reach the best compromise. Some of the newer digital instruments have automatic modes, decreasing fatigue and only boosting amplification when speech is present.

With regard to clarity, remember that hearing aids are <u>aides</u> to hearing. They're not new ears, and they cannot correct for certain limitations in understanding that are more related to severe inner ear distortion, altered brain functioning and poor listening habits. If the hearing aid wearer has cognitive deficits, such as senility or Alzheimer's, the hearing aids may not provide proper communication ability, no matter how well they may be functioning.

Another common limitation of hearing aids is that you may have more difficulty hearing when the sound source is at a distance from you. This occurs, for example, in large conference rooms or auditoriums. Loudness (intensity) decreases as physical distance increases. Unfortunately, most background noise surrounds you, so while the intensity of speech decreases with distance, the intensity of noise may not. This is one reason why hearing aids effectively transmit sound if the speaker talks right into the microphone, but at longer, more realistic distances, reception diminishes. It would be ideal if sound produced at the source transferred directly to you without losing any intensity. It's obviously impractical, however, to ask someone speaking to you to constantly move closer to your ear.

One way to achieve this effect is with direct audio input, where the person speaking holds or wears a microphone. Unfortunately, many hearing aid wearers are reluctant to ask others to use a microphone or wear a wired device. An alternative approach is to use instruments called assistive listening devices that transmit by wireless FM (like a radio), infrared, or induction loop. You may have seen these devices in auditoriums and theaters, and they can be used in combination with your hearing aids. Ask your hearing care professional if the particular hearing aids you are considering will be able to work with these extra features.

"What should I expect with my new hearing aids?"

Hearing aids are not new ears; they're electronic devices; they're not perfect. Since the main goal of amplification is to help communication, recognize that it may take some time to fully adjust to your new hearing. Don't be disappointed if you experience only minimal benefit during the initial trial with amplification. Talk with your hearing professional to determine what you should and shouldn't expect to be able to do when you begin your new life with hearing aids.

The benefit derived from amplification may be subtle. If your new hearing aids ease your daily listening tasks, they're beneficial. Depending on your hearing loss, the goal of the hearing aids may not be to make sounds louder. That is, especially where only high frequency amplification occurs, there are only a few English language sounds in this range (such as /s/, /sh/, /t/, /th/, /f/, and /k/). Therefore, your hearing aids are designed to pick up only these consonants and since we're talking about relatively few sounds, the benefits of amplification may not be readily apparent. It's important to note here that even though we're speaking of a few sounds, these sounds are critically important.

You also need to recognize that prediction of guaranteed long-term benefit from amplification is difficult to determine. A period of initial adjustment and a learning process is required for most new hearing aid users. It may take several weeks before you adjust to the new pattern of sound and learn new "recognition" cues that you probably have not heard for a long time. As a new wearer, you need to be oriented to the world of amplification. You may require a gradual "break-in" wearing schedule (a few hours the first day, six hours the second, nine hours the third, etc.), or you may be encouraged to wear the hearing aids immediately during all your waking hours. You may require additional counseling and training, either individually, or in groups with others with hearing loss, and family members.

You must accept that time is required for adapting to hearing aids. Your ability to understand amplified speech can continue to grow for as long as three months following the use of new hearing aids. Most hearing healthcare professionals will give you a one-month trial period with new hearing aids. If market conditions allow, trial periods may be extended. My advice is, if a trial period is not offered, take your business elsewhere!

It's important that you read the instruction manual that comes with your hearing aids. Hopefully, your provider will have told you everything you need to know about inserting and removing your hearing aids, checking the batteries, cleaning and maintaining the instruments, and using hearing aids with the telephone. But often, too much information can overload the brain! Take the hearing aids home, read the instruction manual, and then call your provider if you have any questions. Then go out and wear them in a variety of listening environments. When you return to your hearing healthcare provider, discuss the situations with which you may have had difficulty so that possible adjustments and fine-tuning can be achieved.

Also remember that hearing aids are sophisticated electronic devices that spend most of their time in a rather unfriendly environment—your ear. Can you imagine what would happen if you placed your home stereo system in a rainforest? Well, your ear canal is somewhat like a rainforest in that it is very warm (about 98.6 degrees), it's moist (with earwax), and it doesn't always receive enough fresh air. As such, hearing aids do require occasional repair. Blockage from earwax is the most common cause for hearing aid malfunction. Ask your hearing aid provider about some of the modern "wax traps" that can help keep earwax out of your hearing aids. You can minimize the need for repair if you are conscientious about cleaning them daily according to instructions and possibly storing them every night in a container that soaks up any excess moisture.

Last, but certainly not least, recognize that hearing is not the same as listening. Hearing simply refers to the audibility of sounds. The purpose of your hearing aids is to provide you with access to the comfortable sounds you've been missing. But listening requires your attention and focus. I'll bet you know of friends (or possibly a family member) who has normal hearing but is a very bad listener. Supplementing your new hearing aids with additional rehabilitation methods such as home-based auditory training, group therapy, speechreading lessons, assistive listening devices, etc., can be very useful in giving you the kinds of communication strategies that can make the difference between understanding and being left out of a conversation, particularly in tough listening environments. Talk to your professional about establishing a comprehensive communication enhancement plan for you.

Conclusions

Now you have the facts, at least as they stand early in the 21st century. Remember, in order to have the best chance of succeeding with hearing aids, be patient with yourself, have a sense of humor, and maintain realistic expectations. You and your brain have consciously and subconsciously created many behaviors to compensate for your hearing loss over the years. Some of the habits you've picked up have probably helped your ability to communicate, but some may have actually impaired your communication skills. Properly fit hearing aids can give you back some of those sounds you've been missing, but you have to learn how to properly use your hearing aids and supplement your "new hearing" with better listening habits. Don't be afraid to call your hearing professional when you have any questions. It's not easy to master all the new features available in hearing aids, so ask for instruction and inform him or her about the aspects of your communication that you're happy with as well as those you still wish to improve.

CHAPTER FOUR
Improving Your Listening And Hearing Skills

Mark Ross, Ph.D.

Dr. Ross received his doctorate at Stanford University. He has worked as a clinical audiologist, a director of a school for the deaf, Director of Research and Training at the League for the Hard of Hearing, and as a Professor of Audiology at the University of Connecticut where he's now a Professor Emeritus. Currently, he is a consultant with the Rehabilitation Engineering Resource Center (RERC) at Gallaudet University in Washington, D.C. Among his activities for the RERC, he writes a bimonthly feature on Developments in Research and Technology for *Hearing Loss: the Journal of Self Help for Hard of Hearing People.* Dr. Ross writes from his experience of having personally worn hearing aids for over 50 years.

I don't know any hard of hearing person who, if a magic wand were available to wave away his or her hearing loss, would not jump at this miraculous opportunity. I know that I would like to be at the head of the line! But life is not a fairy tale and magic wands are in short supply. For most of us with hearing loss, it's simply a pain, one whose impact we're constantly trying to overcome or minimize.

We don't approach the world as "hard of hearing" people, seeking acceptance as a separate social entity. On the contrary, we're trying not to make the hearing loss a defining element of our personal identity; we do this, not by ignoring it, but by striving to reduce its impact in our lives. To realize our goal of continued engagement with the larger society—with our friends, family, jobs, and interests—we employ all the technological tools we can, i.e., hearing aids and other hearing assistive devices. And we use various communication strategies to reduce the inevitable consequences of hearing loss.

By "communication strategies" I mean any activity that might increase your ability to understand speech, either generally or in particular situations, not just technological solutions. Of course technology is a key consideration, but the adjustment process doesn't end there. There are other things you can do to improve your ability to communicate in different situations. When you purchase hearing instruments, you depend upon the hearing healthcare provider's expertise to help in making the proper decision. When it comes to communication strategies and making the best use of all types of hearing technology, <u>you</u> have to take the major responsibility. The concept of personal responsibility for your own action underlies the three recurring themes stressed throughout this chapter: acknowledgment, assertiveness, and communication strategies.

I'll begin this chapter by discussing your personal responsibilities as you strive to improve your hearing capabilities, after which I'll comment on your initial experiences with hearing aids. My focus will be on how you can learn to interpret, enjoy and expand the new world of sound to which you've suddenly been exposed. I'll follow this by discussing speechreading and auditory training exercises that can help you make the most of your residual hearing. Finally, in the last section, I'll present some "hearing tactics," i.e., various kinds of adaptations to real-life situations aimed at improving speech comprehension. In writing this chapter, I've drawn heavily on what I've personally practiced during the many years that I've worn hearing aids. (I shudder to think what my life would be like without them.)

Acknowledgment

The first and indispensable step in practicing effective communication strategies is to accept the reality of the hearing loss. Unless and until you can acknowledge its presence, openly and in a matter of fact way, you're always going to be limited in how effectively you can deal with it. A hearing loss is not something to be ashamed of; it's not a stigma that has to be hidden. <u>Its presence does not diminish you as a human being</u>. By denying or projecting your hearing difficulties onto other people's mouths ("people don't talk as clearly as they used to!"), you fool only yourself. The point is worth emphasizing. The hearing loss is there. Magical thinking, denial, not "wanting to talk about it," will not make it go away. If you don't face up to this reality, unpleasant as it may be, you're condemning yourself to a life of unnecessary stress, anxiety and isolation, as preceding chapters in this book have so beautifully elucidated.

As you know by now, the onset of hearing loss is typically very gradual. What makes this situation particularly difficult for older people is that, initially, they're truly not aware that a hearing loss may be the main reason they're having communication difficulties. They can't very well deny hearing sounds that they're not aware of! This is the point where many of the conflicts between the hard of hearing person and his/her significant others first arise. It's not so much denial as disbelief; they know there are times when they can hear well. After a while, of course, the effects of the hearing loss become apparent to everyone, including the person involved. If these are ignored, then someone can truly be said to be "in denial."

Assertiveness

After you've acknowledged the hearing loss to yourself and to others, you're then in a position to assert your communication needs in various kinds of situations. "Assertiveness" is a concept that underlies many of the specific steps I'll be suggesting later. You must be willing to inform and educate others about what they have to do in order to make it easier for you to hear and understand. It may be as simple as asking the waiter in a restaurant to turn down the background music or to provide you with a written version of the day's selections, or as involved as arranging the seats at a meeting.

Being more assertive about your listening needs by asking others to modify their behavior does not come naturally for many people. It may mean changing the habits of a lifetime, but it can be done and it can be quite liberating (there's got to be some advantage to getting older!). Of course, you don't have to take giant steps in the beginning. Even little ones, as long as you take enough of them, will eventually get you to your goal.

Note that you can be assertive about listening needs without being aggressive or hostile. "Would you mind talking a little louder? I have a hearing loss and that will make it easier for me to understand you," will get better results than, "For Pete's sake, get the mud out of your mouth when you speak to me!" When we assert our hearing needs, we're saying to somebody, "Yes, I really do want to communicate with you."

Communication Exchange

This brings up the third recurring theme in this chapter: both you and the person with whom you're talking are equally involved in a communication exchange. Presumably, this person wants to be understood as much as you want to understand. Unlike a monologue, a conversation is a two-way street. When you suggest that a seating arrangement be modified, or you inform your conversational partners what verbal modifications to make so that you can better understand them, it's as much for their benefit as it is for yours.

What I'm suggesting is that when you work with and help other people communicate more effectively with you, both you and these others benefit. *So, acknowledge your hearing loss, be assertive about your hearing needs, and know that you are a crucial half of any communication interchange.*

Getting the Most out of Your Hearing Aids

As a hard of hearing person you want to ensure that you're making the best use of your residual hearing. This means maximizing the benefit you're receiving through your hearing aids. Amplification is the only "therapy" that directly increases the actual amount of acoustic information available. All the training and practice procedures that will be presented are predicated on you first getting as much useful acoustic information as possible through your hearing aids. Although you ought to realize some immediate benefit from your hearing aids, you should obtain even more help after you get used to them. This requires us to consider both some general principles and some specific practice procedures.

Tenacity

Foremost, don't get discouraged! Remember that while you've had a hearing loss for a number of years and experienced the frustrations of poor hearing, for you the sounds you had been receiving seemed perfectly "normal." Now with hearing aids you're suddenly being exposed to sounds that are not only louder, but a different pattern. You're going to have to reeducate your brain to accept these different sound patterns as "normal." As a rather simple analogy, what you now perceive with hearing aids can be likened to someone talking English with a very different accent. Just as it takes time for an American to get used to, for example, an Australian speaking English, or for a New Englander to comprehend the speech of someone who comes from the Deep South (and vice versa), so it will take some time for you to adjust to the amplified "accent" coming through your hearing aids.

The Adjustment Process

When you first turn on your hearing aids, you're suddenly going to hear many sounds of which you previously were unaware. Many of these sounds will jog familiar memories. For others, you're going to have to consciously identify the source of the sound, either by asking someone or by honing in on it yourself. One woman in a recent hearing aid orientation group was going a little crazy with the hissing and splattering sounds she kept hearing until she realized it was coming from her frying pan. She hadn't heard the sounds of frying food for many years.

Suddenly you're going to be exposed to a world of sound you had forgotten, such as the whirl of the dishwasher, the whine of an electric can opener, the sounds of birds singing, or the "ting" of your microwave when the food is done. Other familiar sounds will be experienced somewhat differently and may even be disturbing, such as traffic noises in the city, the tumult in your favorite restaurant, and the screeching from your grandchildren's boombox (I'm told its music!). It's true that it's a noisy world in which we live, and it seems to be getting noisier all the time. But it's the only world we have and it's the one in which you're going to feel more comfortable when you can more fully hear what's going on. But once you know the cause and source of some unpleasant sound, you can then feel free to ignore it!

Expectations

As you've learned in this book, not everybody will be able to realize the same degree of benefit from hearing aids. After resisting the notion of hearing aids for years, some people when they finally relent expect that hearing aids will recreate their hearing abilities of fifty years ago. It doesn't work that way. While hearing aids will help most people with hearing loss, no matter how advanced a hearing aid or how skilled the hearing care practitioner, the ultimate benefits achievable through amplification are determined by the nature of your auditory disorder. I won't dwell on expectations because it's been well covered in previous chapters, but your satisfaction with hearing aids is going to depend greatly on your expectations, which need to be realistic.

Be in Control

A key in your successful use of hearing aids is working closely with the professionals from whom you received the hearing instruments. They can't give you the full benefits of their skills unless you call upon them with your questions, comments, and experiences. For new hearing aid wearers in particular, the period right after acquiring the hearing aids is crucial. It is at this time that instances of

"Murphy's Law" (whatever can go wrong, will) seem to occur with depressing regularity. Most hearing aid related problems can be solved, or at least minimized, but they won't be if you don't bring them to the attention of your hearing care practitioner. Of all the tales of woe I hear from people regarding their hearing difficulties, unsuccessful attempts to use hearing aids are surely among the most common. It really is a shame; so many people could have been greatly helped and their lives enriched if they had just persisted.

I suggest you wear your hearing aids for as long each day as you feel comfortable, with the eventual goal of wearing them all day every day. But you have to be satisfied that they're helping you hear better and they don't hurt your ears after a few hours. Sometimes, depending upon the nature of what you're hearing, you may want to remove them (e.g., at a hard rock concert, mowing the lawn on a windy day, etc.). Go ahead and take them out and don't feel guilty. Remember—you're the boss. You're in control. They're your ears!

Reeducating the Brain

What "getting used to hearing aids" really means is that you'll be undergoing a learning process. Not only will you have to get used to the hearing aids themselves, but you'll also have to get used to a new pattern of sounds. For some people with long-standing hearing loss, the process of reeducating the brain can be enhanced by specific training or fitting techniques. Because you haven't heard certain sounds for a long time, the signals amplified by the hearing aids may sound strident, artificial, or just downright unpleasant. It's possible that these "unnatural" or "harsh" quality sounds can eventually help you improve your speech perception skills, but only if you can get used to them.

What the hearing aids may be doing is amplifying high frequency speech sounds (like /s/, /sh/ and /f/), elements of which you may not have heard, or have heard differently, for years. Your hearing care practitioner has a good idea of what the final amplification target should be; he or she just can't get there sometimes in one fell swoop. So, don't get discouraged if you're asked to come back for tune-ups. In fact, this may be a mark of an especially conscientious practitioner. Each time you return, your provider may perk up the high frequencies, drop the low frequencies, or do something else to help ease your adjustment to the new auditory experience. While just <u>actively</u> listening to people may be enough to get you used to these new sound sensations, you may also find it helpful to engage in the kinds of "listening" practice procedures that will be presented later.

Speechreading Principles

Until recently, the preferred term for speechreading was lip-reading. We now use speechreading to emphasize the fact that when people talk, a great deal of nonverbal but important information is conveyed via facial and hand gestures, body stance, intonation and rhythm of sentences, and the nature of vocal emphasis placed on words and syllables. For example, the phrase, "<u>Where</u> are you going?" conveys quite a different meaning than "Where are <u>you</u> going. And "CONvict" has quite a different meaning than "conVICT," even though the two words look alike on the lips. Lip movements alone are insufficient to clarify the different meanings in these instances. What speechreading is, then, is lip-reading "plus." Our goal is not only to understand more of what a person is saying by looking at the lips, but also to be attuned to these other important sources of information. While much of this "tuning" may be unconscious, it is nevertheless very real. Speechreading will help you whether you have a mild or profound hearing loss.

If you can see a person's lips and you know the language, then you have already been speechreading—to some extent. I'll bet if I asked you if you can speechread, you'd say, "No!" But you do!

Ask your significant other to silently mouth a month of the year (one of twelve choices). If you can't get it, try a day of the week (that is, seven rather than twelve choices). If you still don't get it (and assuming your partner's lips can be seen clearly—this is very important to check), ask this person to mouth the lip movements for the numbers "three" or "four." Nobody misses this. So, the chances are that to some extent you've already been speechreading, as long as you can observe the lips of the speaker. But you should do even better if you understand the general principles of speechreading.

Visibility

The first general principle is that you must be able to see the lips of the person talking. Now this not only sounds simplistic, but positively insulting! Of course one has to see the lips in order to speechread. But you'd be surprised how many people with hearing loss who need and can benefit from speechreading do not observe the lips of their conversational partners. They may look them "right in the eye" or simply stare off to one side.

The lip movements we're trying to pick up are minuscule, rapid, and very fleeting. Since our vision is most acute at the point of focus, our best chance of perceiving these cues is by looking right at the lips. For example, our peripheral vision should be sufficient to detect facial expressions, hand gestures, body stance, and so forth because they're larger movements. Try it. Look at someone's lips and note that you can also see the expression on his or her face as well as any hand movements.

Think about the implications of these simple rules. You will not be able to speechread when:

- in the dark
- a person's back is turned
- you're far from a person
- your visual acuity is poor (so, pay as much attention to your vision as to your hearing)
- a person's mouth is covered your conversational partner wears a full mustache and beard light is in your eyes
- the face of the person you're talking to is shadowed

In other words, any situation that reduces the visibility of the lips is going to interfere with speechreading. How often have you, or people you know, made an extra effort, perhaps unconsciously, to ensure that you can see the person who's talking? If you have, you've been speechreading, even though you may not have known it.

Restricting Lip Movements

Anything that interferes with movements of the lips is also going to interfere with speechreading. Some people seem unable to talk unless they have a pencil or the frame of eyeglasses jutting out of their mouth. Other people talk as if they were practicing to be ventriloquists—their lips hardly move at all. And some people seem to talk with a perpetual smile, making speechreading almost impossible because of the way the smile distorts lip movements. In a few of these instances, a little assertiveness may help, such as, "Please take the pencil out of your mouth."

But for others it's a losing battle. Because of the wide variations in the size and movement of the lips while talking, there'll be large individual variations in the speechreadability of someone's lips. For people with whom you have a continuing relationship, it's worth reminding them to use more lip movements while talking. Sometimes this works quite well. For the tight-lipped stranger, this may be a futile endeavor. It may be easier to change the world than the way some people talk. So be realistic. You can't win them all.

Familiarity with the Language

You can't speechread unless you know the language. This also sounds quite simplistic, and in a way it is. If you're trying to speechread someone talking in a foreign language, of course you won't be able to. But what this brings up is the notion of predictability. Since only about 30-40 percent of the sounds in the English language are clearly visible on the lips, even in the best of circumstances there are lots of gaps that have to be filled in. This isn't quite as imposing a task as it may appear, as long as you and the person you're talking with share a common language. English is very redundant, with many linguistic and situational cues that can help you correctly predict some words you otherwise couldn't. For example, try filling in the blanks in the following sentences:

    A. Please put the dish on the _____.
    B. He hit a home _____ in the last _____.
    C. Where are you _____?
    D. After dark, it snowed again last _____.
    E. I just heard the weather report. They are _____ a major _____ tonight.

In sentence "A," someone could be saying "floor" or "bookcase," rather than "table," but this is unlikely. Sentence "E" is an example of how a previous sentence (or sentences) can improve predictability. The words are "predicting" and "storm." Now—wasn't that easy?

Native language speakers do this kind of thing unconsciously. No matter what language you've grown up with, you can (or could prior to the onset of your hearing loss) effortlessly understand verbal messages. Don't you often fill in the last part of people's conversations before they finish? This is the kind of predictability I mean. If you're not listening to your native language, then you'll have more difficulty making these predictions (as well as more difficulty understanding speech in noise or other difficult listening situations).

Topic Restrictions

The ability to speechread improves when you can reduce conversational possibilities. When you go to the bank, a municipal office, shop in a clothing store, or talk to a co-worker regarding a particular project, the topics are likely to be limited by the context.

I don't suppose you talk about certificates of deposit in the clothing store, or the weather in Italy at the bank. Basically, "topic restrictions" are another way of employing linguistic predictability.

This is not something you necessarily do consciously. However, the fact that topic restrictions do enter into almost any conversation should make it easier for you to speechread and to keep from making bad guesses. If it makes no sense at all, it probably wasn't the message! Yes, a lot of guessing does take place, and sometimes, as has happened to me, I guess wrong (with occasional embarrassment but just as often, a laugh for everybody). Still, I would rather guess and keep the conversation going than give up.

It's the Message Not the Medium

When you're engaged in conversation, don't focus on speech-reading particular sounds or words. Instead, attend to the message —the meaning of what the other person is trying to convey. If you consciously try to analyze the minuscule, rapid, and fleeting movements of the lips, you're going to be three sentences behind before you figure out the missing sounds or words—if you ever do. Many books on speechreading spend an inordinate amount of time describing how different sounds of speech are made. Speechreading successfully, however, does not require you to identify all the sounds a person forms on his or her lips. What being successful means is that you're able to comprehend what the person is saying.

Because so many of the sounds of speech are either invisible or are formed exactly the same way as other sounds, even the most skilled speechreader cannot identify all of them. What they do, and what you must do, is use your knowledge of the language and your awareness of topic restrictions to fill in the gaps. By focusing on the message rather than specific movements, you'll find that subsequent sentences may clarify words that you may have missed.

Hearing

One crucial principle in speechreading is the necessity for you to use your residual hearing as well as you can. Now, this seems like a contradiction! If we're talking about speechreading, why bring up hearing? Well, how often are you talking to someone while you're not wearing your hearing aids? Maybe late at night or early in the morning, but at most other times you're likely to be wearing them. And why would you not wear them if you know they help you? Normally, then, when conversing with other people, you're going to depend on both speechreading and hearing. And that's fine. Because your goal is to understand speech as well as you can, you should use whatever cues are available to help you realize this goal.

As I mentioned earlier, many of the sounds in English are completely invisible on the lips. For example, look in the mirror while saying the word, "key." It can be said with no movement at all. This is the kind of word that requires context in order to understand.

For example, to the teenager in the house, "No you can't have the _____ to the car!" Context is the only way the word can be understood. Now, while you're still in front of the mirror, silently say the words: /pan/, /ban/, and /man/. They all look alike, don't they? This is where hearing comes in. Fortunately, it's relatively easy to hear the difference between the /b/, /p/, and /m/ sounds, since /b/ is voiced, /p/ is voiceless and /m/ is a nasal sound (also voiced).

In other words, much of what you can't see, you can hear. This is an important principle. It turns out that there are many speech sounds that are very difficult to tell apart visually, and yet are relatively easy to distinguish through hearing (i.e., while the /t/, /d/, and /n/ sounds look identical, they can often be differentiated through hearing). Conversely, other sounds that are difficult to hear (like /s/, /f/, /t/, and /th/) are relatively easy to speechread. So, what we find is that vision and audition provide complementary information. What's lacking or difficult to perceive in one sense can often be picked up in the other. Therefore, depending only on speech-reading, or only on hearing, limits your ability to communicate.

In real life situations, there are always going to be variations in how well you can see and hear someone talking. Noise will tend to mask out many speech sounds and reduce the amount of information you get through hearing. This forces you to depend more on visual cues in order to understand a spoken message. But because the loudness and type of noise constantly vary, these changes will cause your ability to understand speech to vary as well. In some situations you may have to rely almost entirely on vision to understand speech, while in other situations, you may be able to understand even without looking at the speaker. By using both vision and audition as much as possible, and any other sources of information, *most* hard of hearing people can comprehend *most* of what *most* people say in *most* situations. I'm qualifying because there will inevitably be times when you miss part or almost all of a conversation. This will happen. What I'm suggesting is that you think positively. Think of the occasions you can understand rather than the times you can't. That is, think about a half full glass and not a half empty one!

Practice Procedures

Over the years, there has been hundreds of books and articles purporting to teach people how to speechread, often extolling some specific theory and providing lots of practice material. Personally, I find the practice material more helpful than the theories. Practice will help improve just about any skill. I personally had experienced the benefits of intensive speechreading practice several years ago. For about a month I could not use my hearing aids because of an infection in both ear canals. All I could depend upon was speech-reading (with a profound hearing loss in both ears I'm functionally deaf). Ordinarily, I'm a not a very good speechreader, even though I've taken intensive training programs years ago. After several weeks of trying to communicate without hearing, mainly with my wife, I found my ability to speechread her noticeably improving. I still couldn't carry on an extended conversation by speechreading alone, but at least in context I was able to carry on abbreviated conversations. (We did cheat once in a while and use finger spelling to clarify difficult words!) So, with speechreading practice, with and without sound, wherever and with whomever you do it, is going to help you improve your understanding of spoken messages.

Tracking

One creative such exercise, termed tracking procedures, is practiced "live," with a communication partner. Don't be discouraged by the professional jargon. These are basically exercises that require you to comprehend some segment of speech before proceeding to the subsequent segment. In other words, you're required to "track" through a conversation in a sequential manner. The tracking exercises can be structured so they incorporate other training procedures as well. I'll explain how this works.

You're sitting across from your conversational partner. The room is well lit and you're relaxed. (It's going to be fun!) This person has selected a paragraph as practice material; it can be from the newspaper, from a magazine article or book; or specific material related to one's vocation or interests. Whatever material is selected, it's important that the sentences follow each other in some kind of logical sequence. You should be informed of the general content or topic of the paragraph, as would be the case in real life.

Now, while using a soft voice and normal, not exaggerated lip movements (adding noise via television or radio will enhance the realism of the exercise), your partner should read the first sentence of the paragraph to you. Did you get it all? Did you get any of it? Your job is to repeat whatever you understood of the sentence, guessing when you're not sure. You possibly made some errors but also got some words correct.

If you missed any part of the sentence, the first step is for your partner to repeat the whole sentence again, verbatim. You may or may not get it all this time. If not, what your partner has to do is emphasize the parts/words you missed, by making them slightly louder and exaggerating the pronunciation somewhat.

Practicing "Communication Repair" Strategies

In practicing communication repair strategies you're focusing on elements in the communication exchange that have broken down. When you don't understand, the person you're talking to may not know this, or what he or she can do to correct the situation. But you should and so you can advise your conversational partner how to communicate more effectively with you.

The rationale is simple. In conversation, asking "what?" or "huh?" doesn't often help very much. Mostly what people will do when they hear these expressions is to repeat over and over again, maybe just as softly, quickly, or poorly articulated.

Exercises of communication strategies can be helpful. Your task is to try to figure out why you missed what you did, and then to ask your partner to make specific modifications. Maybe the person talked too slowly, or slurred speech, or talked with his or her hands in front of the mouth, or any number of other possibilities. Perhaps you don't need the entire sentence repeated; maybe all you didn't get was the last word. So you ask the person to repeat only the portion you missed. With a creative collaborator, you can simulate many real-life situations.

Your goal is to practice "communication repair" strategies enough in a "protected" situation, so that you feel comfortable in utilizing them everyday. For example, you can ask a ticket agent at an airport to look at you when talking, or to talk a little louder, slower, and so forth. When you assist the person you're talking with to be a more effective communicator with you, you're applying the three themes I spoke about earlier: you're acknowledging your hearing loss, being assertive about your communication needs, and placing equal responsibility for the communication exchange on the person with whom you're talking.

Auditory Training

If we've learned anything in audiology in the past fifty years, it's that the hard of hearing person's perception of speech can be improved with auditory amplification, auditory experiences and auditory training. This has been dramatically illustrated by people with severe to profound hearing loss who have received cochlear implants. Recipients initially report some strange auditory sensations that they're unable to identify or use. After awhile, however, the brain learns to make sense of strange sounds. While new users of hearing aids may not experience anything quite so dramatic, you're sure to discover new sounds in the same world you've been living in for years.

Adaptations of the previously described tracking procedure can serve as helpful "auditory training" procedures. In the auditory version, your partner reads the material for you to repeat while his or her lips are covered (no visual cues). For most people, this is still going to be too easy. Since the most difficult situation for understanding the spoken word is in noise, that is how you should structure a listening situation. Use recorded material, such as books on a CD or tape, as the noise source.

For example, the first sentence is read. If you miss part or all of it, your partner should, in this order:

- repeat it verbatim;
- repeat it—stressing the words you missed;
- if you still miss it, the sentence should be rephrased, but then go back to the original version for you to repeat;
- and finally, let you see and hear the sentence if you still missed it.

After you get the first sentence, your partner should then read the second one and continue the process throughout the entire paragraph. So I suggest no more than 15-30 minutes in the beginning. As you well know, trying to listen under adverse circumstances can be fatiguing.

Self-Administered Training

Getting and keeping a cooperative partner can be quite a challenge. After awhile, you may run out of cooperative partners! Remember, though, the purpose of the training procedure is not to endanger relationships, but to foster good listening habits! You can advance toward the same goal working by yourself, using available CD recordings of books available at libraries. Listen to the recording, initially while following the written version (which requires that the recording be unabridged), and subsequently, when you gain more confidence, you can listen without the help of the script. Listen to the recording for as long you feel comfortable, but I would suggest no less than 15-20 minute sessions three or four times a week. I also suggest that you use a direct audio connection from the player to your hearing aids. This can be with earphones placed over ITC hearing aids, or via the telephone coils and a neckloop or dual silhouette set (see further discussion in Chapter Five).

The purpose of this exercise is twofold: One is to provide you with the experience of listening to the new sounds provided by your hearing aids. It may take time for you to get used to the auditory sensations you're now hearing, but this listening practice will help you realize the goal. Secondly, this gives you confidence that your hearing abilities can be improved with time and practice.

Computer Controlled Home-Based Procedures

There are also training procedures for those people who prefer, or can benefit more, from a more structured training approach. This type of program used to be provided (if at all) by professionals in face-to-face therapy sessions. However, in the past few years, there has been an increasing recognition that the traditional models of auditory and speechreading training are no longer viable, mainly for economic reasons. Face-to-face therapy encounters take time, too much so for traditional third-party payers (Medicare, insurance companies, etc.) to be willing to support. There's clearly a need to develop economically viable methods that are convenient, effective, and relatively inexpensive. In my judgment, two recently introduced self-administered home-based training programs meet these requirements. There are others, but these are the two I've personally tried and am most familiar with. Each comes with a compact disk and a user booklet. Both are user friendly and appear to be based on sound, professional principles (e.g. content, lesson progression, reinforcement, etc.).

Home-Based Training Programs

There are two home-based training programs I would encourage you to consider. The first is "Listening and Communication Enhancement" (LACE), an enhanced auditory training program that includes a variety of listening tasks, supplemented by occasional "helpful hints" regarding effective communication strategies. An explanatory video at the beginning of the program clearly outlines the training procedures. It requires a commitment of some 30 minutes a day, five days a week, for four weeks, although this can be modified somewhat if one wishes. At the conclusion of the program, research studies suggest that speech perception skills can indeed improve. It is recommended that the LACE program be accomplished collaboratively with a referring audiologist, who can remotely monitor your progress.

LACE includes five types of listening tasks, each one beginning at a level where success can be assured; then the program proceeds to more and more difficult listening conditions. Each of the five types of stimuli reflects the kinds of situations and hearing difficulties often reported by people with hearing loss. The first such task requires the comprehension of sentences delivered in noise, probably the most frequently reported challenge. Listeners repeat as much of each sentence as they can. The next screen then presents the sentence visually. If the sentence has been understood ("yes" or "no" buttons on the screen), then the next sentence presentation is made more difficult. If it has not been understood, the sentence is repeated. This basic paradigm is followed for all the subsequent listening tasks. (Further information can be obtained at www.neurotone.com.)

The second home-based training program is "Seeing and Hearing Speech." As the title indicates, visual cues (speechreading) are added to the listening exercises, thus quite nicely complementing the content of LACE. The program consists of four major groups: (1) vowels, (2) consonants, (3) stress, intonation and length, and (4) everyday communications. Each group is broken down into further subgroups and then subdivided further. For example, the consonant group consists of nine subgroups, each of which contains six additional lessons. All in all, it makes for a great deal of practice material on a single CD. The program permits a user to select either the visual or auditory mode, or both together. A variety of speakers present the stimuli, some easier to speechread than others (reflecting what happens in reality).

Users are instantly informed whether they made the right choice. If it's wrong, the user can elect to see or hear the presentation again or just go on to the next stimuli. (Further information can be obtained at www.seeingspeech.com.)

All training procedures, those with partners and those you practice yourself, are designed to improve your communication skills in real life, outside of the practice environment. As long as you're engaged in an effective communication exchange with someone, then you're practicing good "carry-over."

Hearing Tactics

"Hearing tactics" is a term used to describe environmental manipulations that make it easier for you to understand the speech of other people.

Using hearing tactics like military tactics means you must plan ahead, marshal your resources, and engage the "enemy"—the difficult communication situations. No hearing tactic or hearing device, will eliminate all of your hearing problems. But you can take a giant step toward reducing many of them by understanding how you can exert more control over the communicative situation. Next are a few examples.

Move Closer

Always try to move closer to the person talking. This is an underestimated but valuable technique. For example, in the average room, if you're eight feet from someone speaking and you can move to within four feet of this person, you've increased the sound pressure at the microphone of your hearing aids by 6 dB. If you can get within two feet of the speaker, then the increase is 12 dB—a rather significant boost. I really don't recommend getting much closer unless you have a "special relationship" with this individual!

While it's true that some modern hearing aids will compensate for distance by providing more amplification of weaker sounds, and less for the stronger sounds, they will also amplify the background noises in a similar fashion. Better comprehension results when the sound you want to hear is located close to the hearing aid microphone, whether this sound is a person talking, a television set, radio, or anything else. This will improve the speech to noise ratio (the intensity level of the speech relative to the noise) which is perhaps the most important factor underlying your speech perception.

Quiet the Room

This is a principle that applies just about every place you go. When you walk into a restaurant for a relaxing meal and find that the young staff is playing loud music through the P.A. system, what do you do? Here's where assertiveness pays off. Many young people seem completely unaware that there is loud music in the background—this all seems very normal to them. When it's explained to the staff that the music makes speech comprehension virtually impossible for the person with a hearing loss, more often than not they graciously comply with the request to lower the volume.

When you arrive, look for the quietest table. Don't sit in the middle of a room with parties all around you, although you can seat yourself in the center of your group where it's easy for you to see and hear everyone. Stay away from any extra noise-producing areas such as the kitchen, background piano music, an air conditioner or heating system. Better yet, look for places to eat that encourage private conversations; restaurants do differ in their sensitivity to noise.

Many people feel that they have to have the stereo turned on when entertaining people in their home. A gentle reminder to turn it down or even off usually suffices. In a family gathering, the youngsters may have the television set turned up while ignoring it; if it's your house, pull the plug and/or move the youngsters to another room. If it's not your house, try diplomacy or try to move your personal conversation to a quieter area in the house. Whatever environment you happen to be in, make sure you have a good sight-line to all the guests. Don't sit at the end of a long couch. You won't be able to see or hear the person at the other end. If only a small group is involved, try to get some conversational "rules" established. If your social gathering are friends, you can ask that only one person talk at a time. "Cross-conversation" presents one of the most difficult situations for people with hearing loss.

Senior centers and retirement homes, particularly those that serve meals, often present a challenging communication environment. In such places, the acoustical conditions can be improved by:

- acoustical treatment on ceilings and walls;
- rugs, if possible, on the floor;
- or rubber coasters on chair and table legs;
- soft material, such as felt, on dining tables under the table-

cloths to reduce the clattering sounds of dishes and silverware;

• sitting at a smaller (4-person) rather than larger (8-person) table during meals and other activities.

Advance Planning

Plan ahead for any activity. For example, before you attend any large-area listening situation (theater, lecture, house of worship, etc.) call ahead to see if an assistive listening device is available. These devices basically transmit the sound from its source to special receivers (FM radio, infra-red, or the telephone coil in your hearing aid). They enhance the acoustical clarity of sounds that emanate from loudspeakers some distance from you. In other words, they serve as an "acoustical bridge" from the sound source to your ears.

Most such places are required to have such listening devices available, according to the Americans with Disabilities Act (ADA). Houses of worship are an exception, yet many provide such devices as a courtesy. I personally would not attend any large area listening event without ensuring that such devices were available. Without one, I either don't know what's going on or I'm straining so hard to hear that I don't enjoy the activity or performance.

Microphone Technique

Even if assistive listening devices are available in an auditorium, listening problems can still occur, particularly if the sound source comes from someone using a microphone. What I've observed over the years approaches inconsideration by people who should know better when they use a microphone. What seems to happen is that talkers get so wrapped up in what they're saying, they forget that there's a microphone on the podium. Most of these are low-sensitivity microphones, requiring a talker to speak within six inches for effective pick-up. Sometimes, if it's a hand-held microphone, many speakers wave it around as if it were a baton or a pointer— everywhere but close to their mouth. So what do you do?

• You arrive a little earlier and remind the event organizer, the speaker or the minister, of the necessity for the speaker to stay close to the microphone while talking.

• During the talk, some speakers are going to walk away from the microphone still speaking. You ask loudly (but politely) for the speaker to move closer to the microphone.

Other people in the audience will appreciate your assertiveness because of their own hearing difficulty.

- If a lapel instead of a podium microphone is available, ask that it be used and pinned close to the person's mouth.
- If there's a public question and answer period after the talk and you can't hear the questions, don't suffer in silence. Ask for the questions to be repeated before answers are given. Remember that you're probably not the only one in the audience who would benefit.

In a recent hearing aid orientation group, I heard of an excellent example of how a bit of assertiveness can help many other people in the audience. One of the participants complained that he never heard the homilies prepared by the same two women in his church. Their voices were soft and they typically sat two feet or so away from the microphone. Every Sunday, he said he just sat there and waited for them to finish, not understanding a word.

His normal hearing wife then piped up and said, "I never understand them either and I don't think anyone else can!" Before the next service, the husband asked the two women to talk right into the microphone as he was having difficulty understanding them. That Sunday, not only my client, but everyone heard the women loud and clear.

Wrap Up

In this church anecdote, we have an example of the three themes with which I began this chapter. The hard of hearing person had to acknowledge the hearing loss, had to be assertive in approaching speakers, and the effort served the purposes of both parties in the communication exchange. The lesson in this example is that you, as a hard of hearing person, must be more than a passive recipient of hearing "services." You have to take more control over your own listening needs. Work closely with your hearing healthcare professionals. They have information and skills that will help you.

No—magic wands are not available to "wave" away your hearing loss, but with the appropriate use of modern technology and the judicious use of appropriate communication strategies, you can go a long way in reducing the impact hearing loss is having in your life.

CHAPTER FIVE
Assistive Technology
Secrets to Better Hearing

Douglas L. Beck, AuD

Dr. Beck earned his Master's Degree from the State University of New York at Buffalo (1984) and his doctorate from the University of Florida at Gainesville (2000). His career started at the House Ear Institute (Los Angeles) in cochlear implant research and intraoperative cranial nerve monitoring. Five years later he was appointed Assistant Professor of Otolaryngology and Director of Audiology at Saint Louis University. Eight years later he co-founded a private audiology-based dispensing practice. In 1999, Dr. Beck was appointed as Editor-In-Chief for www.audiologyonline.com, www.speechpathology.com and www.healthyhearing.com. He joined Oticon in 2005 as Director of Professional Relations. In 2008, he was appointed Web Content Editor for the American Academy of Audiology. Dr. Beck is a prolific author and has addressed a wide variety of audiology and professional topics via hundreds of publications.

Chapter Five is added courtesy of Oticon, Inc.

Introduction

The multiple benefits of advanced binaural hearing aids are tremendous. Not only do modern hearing aids improve our ability to hear and listen, but they improve the quality of life for those who wear them. Nonetheless, it is important to keep in mind that hearing aids are primarily designed to enhance the sounds of conversational speech. In particular, hearing aids are maximally beneficial when people are speaking in a relatively or nearly quiet acoustic environment. Although modern advances such as digital noise reduction circuits and adaptive directionality help the hearing aid wearer hear better and more comfortably, sometimes additional help is needed in very challenging listening situations. In particular, for people with hearing loss, the number one complaint with and without hearing aids is "understanding speech in noise."

Unfortunately, as one might suspect, the "noise" people complain about most often is the sound of *other* people speaking! For example, let's consider some very common situations.

Imagine you're at an extremely popular crowded and noisy restaurant. Sometimes the person you'd like to attend to is right next to you (on your left or right) or perhaps sitting across the table. You might want to say a quick "hello" to a friend passing by or perhaps sitting two tables away. You might also need to converse with the waiter or want to listen to the music through the public address system. All of these sound sources represent things you'd like to be able to listen to comfortably—one at a time. However, in this (and every other) crowded restaurant, people often speak at *exactly* the same time, making it very difficult for anyone to understand!

Next, imagine you have excellent hearing and you're speaking with a good friend while attending a noisy cocktail party. Suddenly, you hear your name spoken by someone behind you. What would happen? You would very likely be able to immediately focus your listening ability directly on the person that spoke your name. That is, when normally hearing ears send an important signal to our brain, the brain can quite often "focus" on the *one voice* in the noisy crowd that spoke your name. As long as both ears are working normally and supply the brain with the full complement of acoustic cues, the brain has a tremendous capacity to focus on sounds and voices of maximal interest while minimizing (that is, dismissing) inconsequential sounds with little or no meaning.

The human brain is the most sophisticated processor on the planet, and it needs *all* of the acoustic cues available (loudness, timing, left versus right, pitch and more) to make maximal sense of speech in noise. There remains a vast difference between the world's fastest and best information processor (the human brain) and the amazing technology in the very best hearing aids. Simply stated, hearing aids don't know who *you* prefer to pay attention to, while the human brain knows exactly what to do and can selectively focus attention and effort on the voice (or sound) of interest within milliseconds. As a result, hearing aids may amplify multiple voices at the same time so that people wearing hearing aids may sometimes hear way too much human speech in noisy restaurants, cocktail parties, ballparks, weddings, celebrations and other noisy environments. These situations can be difficult and frustrating. Naturally, some people blame their hearing aids, but the hearing aid's first job is to make sounds louder.

At the time of this writing (2011), many hearing aids have the ability to go beyond simply making sounds louder. That is, some hearing aids can better preserve spatial cues, loudness differences and important high frequency information far better than ever before, thereby providing more accurate representation of the sounds around us. However, not all hearing aids have these advanced features. For more information on advanced features, please visit: www.oticonusa.com

Advanced Concepts in Assistive Technology

There are many types of assistive devices that can be used with and without hearing aids. These supplement sound delivery from sound sources we choose to listen to in difficult and challenging listening situations. New technology has facilitated wireless solutions to specifically address (and solve) the three most common "problem areas" for hearing aid wearers: understanding speech in noise; using the telephone; and listening to television.

Fortunately, advanced *connectivity* solutions for hearing aid wearers helps bridge the gap between virtually all sound sources. Connectivity solutions help people listen in challenging acoustic environments such as during use of the telephone, television, DVDs, CDs, MP3s and more (see glossary at end for acronym definitions).

Connectivity

Connectivity can be grossly defined as "the state of being connected."[1] However, of greater importance and with specific regard to hearing aids and amplification, connectivity is all about *connecting people to each other.* Over the last three or four years, connectivity-based hearing products have become increasingly available to provide seamless, easy-to-use and compatible solutions, all designed to be used with advanced hearing aids. Connectivity products available in 2011 and 2012 have been designed to work with advanced hearing aids to make listening easier, more comfortable, successful and more enjoyable, even in the most challenging hearing environments. Further, and of significant importance, hearing aids and other connectivity devices have been shown to clearly improve the quality of life for the wearer[2].

Technology Notes

In general, connectivity products use Bluetooth technology. Although a thorough explanation of Bluetooth is beyond the scope of this section, the primary "take home" point is that Bluetooth technology can provide a wireless (radio wave) connection to virtually *any* sound source. Unfortunately, Bluetooth technology cannot easily be incorporated directly into tiny and discreet hearing aids because Bluetooth circuits are large and would increase the size of the hearing aid, and Bluetooth circuits consume significant electric power, which would significantly reduce the battery life of the hearing aid. To learn more about Bluetooth, please visit: http://www.howstuffworks.com/bluetooth.htm.

Nonetheless, one excellent and practical solution that allows use of Bluetooth technology has been the development of "gateway" devices, such as the Oticon Streamer (Figure 5-1). Gateway devices serve as a power source and control unit to accept the Bluetooth signal from any sound source and convert it into a magnetic wireless signal that the hearing aids can process in virtually real time.

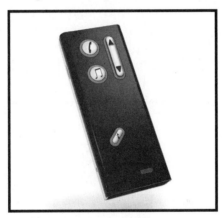

Figure 5-1: the Oticon Streamer

The Oticon Streamer allows the wearer to turn their hearing aids into a hands-free headset. Specifically, the Oticon ConnectLine System allows Bluetooth (and direct connect) transmission from *any* sound source to be sent to the Streamer. The Streamer, in turn, sends a wireless signal to both advanced hearing aids simultaneously.

To learn more about Bluetooth and Connectivity, please visit: http://www.oticonusa.com/Oticon/Professionals/Connectivity.html

Three Connectivity-Based Assistive Technologies

The three most applicable connectivity-based technologies are:
- ConnectLine Microphone
- ConnectLine TV Adapter
- ConnectLine Telephone Adapter

ConnectLine Microphone

The ConnectLine Microphone is a discreet clip-on microphone designed to pick up and transmit a companion's voice while reducing the negative impact of distance and background noise (Figure 5-2). It is small, measuring approximately 1 inch by 2 inches by ½ inch and weighs 13 grams. The ConnectLine Microphone wirelessly transmits a Bluetooth signal to the Oticon Streamer across distances of up to 40 feet. The Streamer then sends a wireless signal to the hearing aids. For hearing aid wearers, the wireless transmission from the ConnectLine Microphone to the hearing instruments means an enhanced ability to engage in challenging acoustic situations such as one-on-one conversations in noisy restaurants, cocktail parties and while riding in a car. Additionally, the ConnectLine Microphone helps minimize or remove sound distortions due to reverberant environments (e.g., as might be evident in large halls and houses of worship). ConnectLine Microphone preserves sound quality and an enhanced signal-to-noise ratio from a greater distance (up to 40 feet) than one would expect with traditional hearing aid microphones.

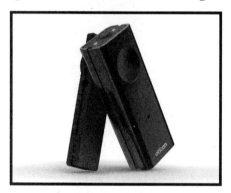

Figure 5-2: the OticonConnectLine Mic

The ConnectLine Microphone is worn (or hand held) by the person speaking, thereby allowing the wearer to hear the other person's voice directly through their hearing aids. The ConnectLine Microphone allows the wearer to experience reduced background noise (as compared to using their hearing aids in a noisy environment), reduced reverberation (echo) and an improved signal-to-noise ratio, since the person speaking is generally within inches of the ConnectLine Microphone.

For more information about the ConnectLine Microphone, please visit: http://www.hearingreview.com/issues/articles/2011-03_04.asp

ConnectLine TV Adapter

The ConnectLine TV Adapter (Figure 5-3) is small, approximately 3 inches square, and unobtrusive. It easily connects to the "audio output" of any TV and runs on its own power supply. Of course, some older television models (20 or more years old) may not not have an "audio output." Fortunately, a simple microphone can be attached (via tape or Velcro) to the TV's speaker to pick up the sound. The ConnectLine TV Adapter sends a Bluetooth signal to the Oticon Streamer with a push of the button and connects automatically whenever the Streamer is activated. While using the ConnectLine TV Adapter, wearers listen through their hearing aids at their preferred volume level and without the "latency delays" that are common in off-the-shelf Bluetooth transmitters. There is no need for recharging and no additional gadgets or loop installations when using the ConnectLine TV Adapter. The TV Adapter is readily managed via the Streamer's easy-to-use button controls and can transmit up to thirty feet.

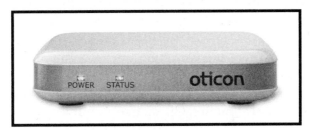

Figure 5-3: the OticonConnectLine TV Adapter

ConnectLine Telephone Adapter

Telephone use is a matter of personal choice and is critically important for safety, communication and to enhance connectivity. Many seniors do not want to learn how to use a new phone despite having difficulties hearing when they use their current phone. The ConnectLine Phone Adapter (Figure 5-4, next page) overcomes this problem by turning *any* existing landline phone into a Bluetooth phone. The ConnectLine Telephone Adapter sends a Bluetooth signal to the Streamer at the push of a button and connects automatically whenever the phone is activated.

It has also been noted[3] that traditional telephone coils and loops systems do not always provide superior speech recognition due to hearing aid (and earmold) vent size, background noise, electromagnetic interference, and sometimes, even the physical positioning of the telecoil and telephone can be problematic. Further, these researchers reported when both ears were used *simultaneously* while listening via telephone, significant improvements in speech recognition occurred.

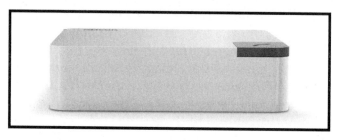

Figure 5-4: the OticonConnectLine Phone Adapter

Indeed, the ConnectLine Phone Adapter transmits the Bluetooth signal up to 30 feet and the Streamer sends the signal to both ears simultaneously—thus facilitating easier telephone conversations.

Summary

Advanced binaural hearing aids improve the quality of life for those who wear them. However, hearing aids are maximally beneficial when people are speaking in relatively quiet, or nearly quiet acoustic environments. Often, in difficult and very challenging listening situations, assistive technologies designed to be used with advanced hearing aids are of significant value and benefit. Oticon's ConnectLine System combines the Streamer with the ConnectLine Microphone, TV Adapter and Telephone Adapter to allow simple, elegant, seamless and affordable solutions for the most demanding listening situations.

References, Recommended Readings and Websites

1. Beck DL and Fabry D. (2011) Access America—it's about connectivity. *Audiology Today* 22(1):24-31.

2. Beck DL and Harvey M. (2009) Creating successful professional-patient relationships. *Audiology Today* 21(5):36-47.

3. Picou EM and Ricketts TA. (2011) Comparison of wireless and acoustic hearing aid-based telephone listening strategies. *Ear and Hearing* 32(2):209-220.

Recommended Reading

Beck DL and Holmberg M. (2011) Connectivity in 2011—enhancing the human experience, *The Hearing Review 18* (3):38,69-70 [http://www. hearingreview.com/issues/articles/2011-03_04.asp].

Recommended Websites

- www.oticonusa.com
- http://www.howstuffworks.com/bluetooth.htm
- http://www.oticonusa.com/Oticon/Professionals/Connectivity .html
- http://www.hearingreview.com/issues/articles/2011-03_04.asp

Glossary of Acronyms (this chapter)

AT (Assistive Technology): broad term for devices and equipment for persons with hearing loss that provide improved ability to hear

BTE (Behind-The-Ear): a hearing aid style that sits behind the ear

CIC (Completely-In-the-Canal): a hearing aid style that sits in the canal closest to the eardrum

EM (Electromagnet, Electromagnetic): an iron core surrounded by a coil of wire; an EM field is used for transferring sound in AT devices

FM (Frequency Modulation): variation of the instantaneous frequency of a carrier wave in accordance with the signal to be transmitted; commonly used in assistive technology devices

ITE (In-The-Ear): a hearing aid style that sits in the canal and bowl of the ear

MP3 (MPEG Audio Layer 3): a digital audio encoding format using a form of lossy data compression; common usage plays and stores music, no larger than a pack of cigarettes

Appendix I
Hearing Loss—Degrees and Types

The degree of hearing loss you experience—that is, how much loss at various frequencies—will often determine the degree of difficulty you'll have. It's also influenced by where the hearing loss appears. For example, if you have significant loss of hearing in the high frequencies, but you hear perfectly in the lower range for speech reception, you'll miss many of the corresponding high frequency consonant sounds such as /s/, /sh/, /t/ and /th/. On the other hand, if you have the same degree of loss, but in the lows, and you hear perfectly in the high range, your difficulty will be hearing the corresponding low frequencies that happen to include all the vowels sounds.

Intelligibility for speech comes mostly from the higher frequencies. The lower frequencies carry the *power* for speech. Therefore, the amount of hearing loss at different frequencies determines the challenges you will face with your hearing loss and hearing aids. Another very important factor is your speech comprehension ability under ideal conditions as well as background noise. Your hearing healthcare practitioner will make these assessments and determinations in order to make the most ideal hearing aid selection.

If you have only a low frequency hearing loss and sounds are made louder (everything else considered normal), you should hear quite well. On the other hand, without use of hearing aids, the brain finds it very challenging to interpret high frequency sounds that have been made louder because you may only need a very narrow (or very broad) range louder. If all the high frequencies are amplified (not by using hearing aids but by shouting) when you only need a narrower range made louder, it will typically add to distortion and discomfort. Therefore, you might now better understand how fitting hearing aids is a tricky, delicate and highly scientific business.

Generally speaking, there are only two basic types of hearing loss: *sensorineural* or *conductive*. You could also have a combination of both. A conductive loss suggests a mechanical problem. That is, you might have earwax in the outer canal plugging the ear and preventing sound transmission. Or you could have fluid in the middle ear, common in children, also preventing transmission of sound. Conductive hearing losses are usually an easy fix by removing or treating the cause. Upon successful treatment, hearing is usually restored to normal.

However, sensorineural hearing loss is quite another matter. As the name implies, if the problem is in the sensory apparatus or neurological process, it is quite rare to return hearing to normal without some kind of mechanical intervention such as a cochlear implant or hearing aids.

There are about six general ranges of hearing loss that we refer to in audiology practice. Each poses its own inherent problems both in hearing as well as hearing aid fitting. Usually, the greater the loss of hearing, the greater the power you will need in a hearing aids.

The range of hearing losses include:

- **normal** hearing, 0-20 dB
- **mild** hearing loss, 21-40 dB
- **moderate** loss, 41-55 dB
- **moderate-severe** loss, 56-70 dB
- **severe** loss, 71-90 dB
- **profound** loss is greater than 90 dB

The decibel (dB) is a unit of sound pressure while frequency is the number of vibrations that occur in a sound wave. Together, they make up the audiogram and can give you a pictorial representation of your hearing or hearing loss. As mentioned earlier, it isn't just the degree of hearing loss that matters, where it is—low, mid, high range—will determine your hearing challenges.

Appendix II
Hearing Care Professionals

Audiologists are trained to perform routine and highly technical diagnostic tests to determine what is causing abnormal auditory function. They have a depth of understanding of the physiology, neurology, anatomy and pathology of the auditory system because of their required education. Also, they provide rehabilitation to those with hearing loss ranging in degrees from mild to profound. Over the past few decades the field of audiology has expanded to include the assessment of hearing loss for the purpose of selecting and fitting hearing aids. Today, the Doctor of Audiology Degree (Au.D.) is designed to emphasize the diagnostic and clinical skills needed to manage a private practice not unlike the medical professional, and to enhance clinical skills, including hearing aid dispensing.

Hearing Instrument Specialists can dispense hearing aids without the requirement of college or university education. Their training is managed through licensing and state requirements to assure they are knowledgeable and capable of performing necessary measurements for the selection and fitting of hearing aids. They can pursue additional training to achieve Board Certification (BC). In order for members to be board certified, a written examination must be taken and passed. This examination is more demanding of specific knowledge than is the examination of individual states. In order to obtain maximum objectivity, the national board examination process is managed by a highly knowledgable group of experts.

Index